PSYCHIATRY IN CRISIS

PSYCHIATRY IN CRISIS

Edited by

Richard C. W. Hall, M.D.

Department of Psychiatry and Medicine
Medical College of Wisconsin
Milwaukee, Wisconsin

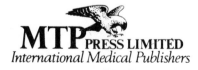
MTP PRESS LIMITED
International Medical Publishers

Published in the UK and Europe by
MTP Press Limited
Falcon House
Lancaster, England

Published in the US by
SPECTRUM PUBLICATIONS, INC.
175-20 Wexford Terrace
Jamaica, N.Y. 11432

ISBN: 0-85200-576-8

Printed in the United States

*Dedicated to my Parents
and Senior Citizens Everywhere*

ACKNOWLEDGEMENT

I would like to gratefully acknowledge the contributions of Mrs. Mary Ellen Voegtline and Mrs. Dorothy Manley for their assistance and preparation of these manuscripts.

CONTRIBUTORS

RICHARD DeVAUL, M.D.
Department of Psychiatry and
 Behavioral Sciences
University of Texas Medical
 School at Houston
Houston, Texas

NEIL B. EDWARDS, M.D.
Department of Psychiatry
University of Tennessee Center
 for the Health Sciences
Memphis, Tennessee

JEROME D. FRANK, M.D.
Department of Psychiatry
John Hopkins University
Baltimore, Maryland

EARL R. GARDNER, Ph.D.
Department of Psychiatry
Medical College of Wisconsin
Milwaukee, Wisconsin

EUGENIA L. GULLICK, Ph.D.
Department of Psychiatry and
 Mental Health Sciences
Medical College of Wisconsin
Milwaukee County Mental
 Health Complex
Milwaukee, Wisconsin

RICHARD C.W. HALL, M.D.
Department of Psychiatry
 and Medicine
Medical College of Wisconsin
Milwaukee, Wisconsin

ALVIN J. LEVENSON, M.D.
Department of Psychiatry and
 Behavioral Sciences
University of Texas Medical
 School at Houston
Houston, Texas

THOMAS B. MACKENZIE, M.D.
Departments of Psychiatry
 and Medicine
University of Minnesota
 Medical School
Minneapolis, Minnesota

DAVID B. MARCOTTE, M.D.
Department of Psychiatry and
 Mental Health Sciences
Milwaukee County Mental
 Health Complex
Medical College of Wisconsin
Milwaukee, Wisconsin

CHESTER M. PIERCE, M.D.
Harvard University
Cambridge, Massachusetts

MICHAEL K. POPKIN, M.D.
Departments of Psychiatry
 and Medicine
University of Minnesota
 Medical School
Minneapolis, Minnesota

JONAS R. RAPPEPORT, M.D.
Department of Psychiatry
Institute of Psychiatry and
 Human Behavior
University of Maryland School
 of Medicine
Baltimore, Maryland

DANIEL A. SEARING, J.D.
U.S. Department of Justice
Civil Rights Division
Washington, D.C.

EARL SHELP, Ph.D.
Institute of Religion
Baylor College of Medicine
Texas Medical Center
University of Texas Health
 Science Center
Houston, Texas

HERZL R. SPIRO, Ph.D.
Department of Psychiatry and
 Mental Health Sciences
Medical College of Wisconsin
Milwaukee, Wisconsin

WILLIAM TAYLOR III, ESQUIRE
Zuckerman, Spaeder, Taylor
 and Kolker
Washington, D.C.

JUDY BAGGETT THRASHER, M.I.J.
St. Luke's Episcopal Hospital
Texas Medical Center
Houston, Texas

WILLIAM L. WEBB, JR., M.D.
Department of Psychiatry
University of Tennessee Center
 for the Health Sciences
Memphis, Tennessee

SIDNEY ZISOOK, M.D.
Department of Psychiatry and
 Behavioral Sciences
University of Texas Medical
 School at Houston
Houston, Texas

Contents

1
Psychiatry: Is Our Hour Up?

Richard C.W. Hall

"Enough," he shouted at his analyst. "Enough psychiatrists! I can't stand it any longer. When I graduated from residency 20 years ago, I thought I could help my patients, be a doctor, and be respected by my colleagues. Now I feel that I've wasted my life."

"It's about your father's expectations," his analyst said knowingly, writing on his pad.

The doctor-patient responded in the affirmative. "Yes, my father wanted me to be a success. He respected knowledge, and the compassion of a physician who cared for his patient. He had a need for me to be admired and I wanted to fulfill that need! Now you tell me that what I am upset about is not the fact that my profession has fallen into disrepute and is the subject of attack, that I no longer know how to practice medicine, that my colleagues no longer hold me in esteem, that my patients are contemptuous of me, that I am being sued, that all the things that I learned are no longer felt to be true, that the medical model is no longer a good one for psychiatry, that my training makes me no better than a lay person, that all my ideas of disease are wrong, that the conditions that I have been treating for years are adaptive processes, that medical schools wish to take psychiatry from their curriculum, or that the government says that there is no place for my specialty. No, what I am really upset about, according to you, is that my father would not be proud of what I'm doing. Can't you see that I'm not proud of what I'm doing?"

"Aha! Do you see?" said the analyst. "Your need to please your father is what's making you unhappy now!"

"Aha!" said the doctor-patient back. "Do you see that you are a pompous fool and that I dislike you intensely? Do you see that I dislike your arrogance and your self-professed omnipotence? And do you see that I am contemptuous of you for not listening to what I have to say?"

Note: This chapter is an expanded version of a paper published in Psychiatric Opinion (Hall, 1979); parts reproduced with permission.

> "But that," said the analyst, smiling at the doctor-
> patient, "is the product of transference. Your hour
> is up."

Is our hour up? Have we, in fact, taken on all of the attributes of
the arrogant and grandiose psychotherapist depicted above, as well as
those of his outraged patient? What is the reality of our concern? What
is our future? The chapters that follow will highlight many of psychiatry's
current conflicts. Our purpose is to trace, at least in part, how we have
reached our current position and, more important, to suggest remedies
for the future. Let us, to paraphrase Churchill, hope that psychiatry's
hour is not yet up, but rather that we are just beginning our finest
hour, that this is not the beginning of the end, but rather just the end
of the beginning.

Throughout the history of medicine, psychiatrists have been somewhat
different from their colleagues. We have a long tradition of being "alien-
ists." And yet, during the last 80 years, psychiatry has been accepted
by both the public and the medical profession. During this time, it has
developed a strong scientific underpinning and accomplished great good.
Psychiatry has become part of the curriculum of every medical school in
the country, has met severe national needs for increased mental health
care following the first and second world wars, and has been creative in
developing new research and treatment approaches. The advent of neuro-
leptics during the 1950s, the increased interest in somatopsychic and
psychosomatic medicine, the development of effective treatment programs,
as well as the decline in the numbers of patients committed long-term to
state psychiatric facilities have all enhanced the image of psychiatry.
Thus, it cannot be argued that our current crisis is the result of a credibility gap produced by either sterility or stagnation. Rather, our crisis
stems from public fear of mind control and of psychiatrists colluding with
governmental agencies, from role diffusion, and from a series of internal
and external assaults that have affected our credibility. We are being
rent asunder from within and without, and therein lies the danger. Psychiatry must be a field that not only tolerates, but encourages, a diversity
of opinion. However, one can raise questions as to the boundaries that
these opinions take in the name of science. Here, I believe, is where we
have become vulnerable. How have we reached our current state? What
forces have worked upon us? How might we change our future?

OUR HISTORICAL DEVELOPMENT

Two hundred years ago, when psychiatry was first recognized as a
medical specialty, the function of the psychiatrist was to care for the
hospitalized insane. Mental hospitals had gradually become warehouses
for segregating the undesirable. Often they were staffed by less than
successful physicians. The abuses that took place in these facilities
finally resulted in a public outcry for improved care of the mentally ill.
While the rest of medicine moved dramatically forward, psychiatry continued in its caretaker role. Following World War I, when psychiatric
casualties became a matter of serious national concern, psychiatry began
to exert innovative leadership, developing new social programs and treatment models. By the 1930s, psychiatry was ensconced to the point that
the analytic concept of neurosis was well accepted by the medical profession. Once this theory gained acceptance, it became an easy matter to
apply it to society as a whole. Psychoanalytic intervention aimed at cor-
recting societal ills became commonplace. Analysts, politicians, the intel-
ligentsia, and the public alike awaited spectacular results based upon a
deluge of early promises. Although the promises were numerous, societal

improvements were few and far between. The whole oversold concept of primary prevention withered on the vine. Psychoanalysts became increasingly grandiose in their delusion of being able to apply analytic theories to social problems. These delusions culminated in offers to provide services to political leaders, and finally in suggestions that the way to achieve world peace was to require that political leaders be analysed (Frank, 1977a).

Following the second world war, when the number of psychiatric casualties was fully appreciated, the government began to lavish support on psychiatry for training, research, and practice. New training programs abounded and rapidly produced a sizable number of practicing psychiatrists. These new psychiatrists, who believed many of the myths of the past, heeded the government's cries for more "outreach and contact" by becoming "team leaders" and enlisting ever-growing numbers of paraprofessionals and nonprofessionals to carry out their treatment orders. All interventions by their "team" were deemed appropriate and therapeutic, since they were provided under the direction of the psychiatrist. Soon, however, the public need for psychotherapists to serve in Veterans' Administration hospitals and community mental health centers was filled by this newly created, nonpsychiatric manpower. Initially, the majority of these organizations wished to have psychiatrists administrate their programs. However, they "settled" for nonpsychiatrists when no MDs came forth to accept the jobs. This "settlement" produced strong social forces to license and certify nonmedical psychotherapists. At the same time, "new therapies" were emerging. Transactionalists, existentialists, Gestaltists, behavioralists, Rolffers, regressive therapists, and so on, all staked out new claims for improving the mind. The establishment and acceptance of these new schools, which required no medical training, produced drastic changes in the mental health profession. A doctrine of "professional egalitarianism" emerged, which was defined by Eaton (1977) as "the notion that everyone can do almost everything − all it takes is a warm heart and extended hand." Psychiatry had abrogated its leadership role. Psychotherapy was no longer seen as a medical skill. Psychology, social work, and nursing all accepted psychiatry's invitation to assume power. As the independence and political support for these disciplines grew, so did the antagonisms between them and psychiatry. Members of our own field increased the public's concern and confusion by suggesting that not only was mental illness a myth (Szasz, 1961; Laing and Esterson, 1964), but that those who purported to cure it were either self-deceived or deceiving the public. Such statements, widely touted by the lay press, suggested that the profession was thereby staffed by either charlatans or fools for, if doctors had good motivation and intent but carried out useless work, they were fools; if they did their work falsely and only for profit, they were charlatans.

Lewis-Harris polls taken at this time showed that as many as 80% of the American public were unaware of the differences between psychiatrists and psychologists. More than half of our medical colleagues were reported to believe that psychiatrists had no special skills that could not be assumed by other medical disciplines. Devisiveness within the ranks of psychiatry, based on the clinician's respective orientation or school, continued, with each group of practitioners discrediting their colleagues while claiming to have the answer for understanding and treating mental illness. The press continually called attention to the abysmal lack of statistical and scientific proof defining the effectiveness of our treatments. Judd Marmor (1979) suggested that three revolutions in psychotherapy had created this situation. The Freudian approach to analysis, the first revolution, initiated the scientific approach to the cognitive study of behavior. This was followed by the formation of behavioralistic schools, which rejected cognitive and suggestive therapeutic concepts and focused on observable behavior and techniques for modifying it. Behavioralism was replaced by the school of experimental or new therapies, such as Rolffing, tickling, age regression, and so on, which developed during the late 60s and 70s. These schools rejected both the cognitive and behavioral models and were seen by Marmor (1978) as reflecting "the deepening revolution against scientific technology and what it has brought. In general, there was an anti-intellectualism, a loss of faith in conventional values, in the materialism inherent in the scientific and technical community. There existed a distrust of and rebellion against authority; feelings of loneliness within a crowd; a sense of loss of community; and a search for things beyond the material world. The new therapies were seen as offering salvation to those who wished for self-acceptance without facing the dilemma of self-change; a cure without dealing with the reality of one's problems. The new therapies were 'packaged' to provide a synthetic and instant intimacy and were thus seen as a painless remedy for loneliness." If Marmor is correct in his analysis of the goals of these new therapies, one must question their use by orthodox psychiatrists, yet this is what happened. The marketplace, rather than scientific fact or professional concern, determined how we practiced our discipline. When we began to "sell" the new fad therapies, we tarnished our credibility. Perhaps our medical colleagues were not far wrong when they suggested that psychiatry was moving away from its scientific foundations in medicine.

The public's perception of psychiatry began to change significantly during the late 60s and early 70s. The Vietnamese war and the counterculture movements of those times produced strong antiscientific feelings. Professional organizations and science were seen by many as part of a politically controlled, military/industrial complex. The abuses of psychiatric research by governmental agencies, which received widespread coverage in the press, further eroded the credibility of psychiatry as a patient advocate and produced new fears of government mind control. As Allen Stone (1976) has commented, "The American public was fearful of a therapeutic state, a clockwork orange vision of citizens drugged and bugged by the psychiatric establishment." These fears united the far right and left, who shared the nightmare of political mind control centers run by a few "Doctor Strangeloves" who were themselves under governmental control. The public was presented with an image of psychiatry (e.g., "One Flew Over the Cuckoo's Nest," "Madness in Medicine," and "The Outrage of Psychiatry") as a brutal and coersive discipline — an image that did little to diminish the public's skepticism or suspicion of psychiatrists. These negative images helped produce new groups of social champions whose self-proclaimed job it was to protect the mentally ill from the abuses of psychiatry. These groups were all too willingly joined by psychologists, social workers, and ministers who practiced therapy. Since they were nonmedical practitioners, they could not be accused of drugging or altering brain function through ECT or psychosurgery. They provided a humanistic treatment while psychiatrists raped the mind. A new jihad began, each side fighting the other with divine guidance. Both the medical and nonmedical psychotherapists knew their cause was just and that they could win only by totally destroying the enemy. No negotiated peace was possible. The war followed Colemen's (1957) doctrine that one must regard one's opponents with hostility and gain one's viewpoint at all costs. Success could be complete only if the opponent was ruined in the process.

The struggle between medical and nonmedical therapists moved rapidly to the political arena. Unfortunately, psychiatry seemed slower than other disciplines to make its fight public. Allen Stone (1979), speaking on "The Future of American Psychiatry Under Law," took organized psychiatry to task when he said that it had paid a "significant price for its failure to participate in such landmark decisions as the Wyatt-Stickney Case, the first great class action, right to treatment litigation." "Right to treatment litigation has been successfully pursued all over the country and organized psychiatry has missed the opportunity to take the initiative and to shape the legal precedents which implement that right." "Organized psychiatry continued its myopic policies" when the APA had the opportunity to enter the Wyatt case and declined. "There, the litigating attorneys were joined by the Justice Department, the American Psychological Association, the National Association for Mental Health, indeed, every significant group interested in the mentally disabled, except the American Psychiatric Association." This is but one example of a situation in which organized psychiatry had a clearly formulated position but failed to act in its own best interest.

Other organizations were less hesitant to use their organized political muscle. The American Psychological Association, for example, recently announced that Governor Brown of California had signed into law State Bill 259, which "authorized health facilities on local determination to grant staff membership, clinical privileges, or both, to licensed psychologists meeting prescribed requirements as defined by state law." The American Psychological Association proudly noted that this legislation protected health facilities that elect to extend staff or clinical privileges to psychologists. The legislation, it should be parenthetically noted, was introduced by California State Senator Paul Carpenter, who is a psychologist as well as a member of the legislature (APA News, 1978).

Psychiatry's movement from the medical model had become so prevalent that many leaders in the field began to question its ability to recover. More important, some, such as Treffert (1978), suggested that the erosion of confidence in psychiatry had become so severe as to deter patients from seeking treatment. "Now, having tremendously successful treatment tools, psychiatry finds itself with eroding credibility; still, with responsibility for sizable numbers of patients, but without opportunity to use, and even with specific prohibition against using, those tools."

Herman Denber (1978) raises similar concerns when he traces the decline of psychiatry in a somewhat different way, seeing the inception of the sector system in France and the implementation of the team concept in Great Britain as fostering the development of the community mental health movement in the United States. This latter movement, which was founded in the hope of providing great public good, may have in fact caused harm by depopulating state hospitals of patients in need of care; by reducing government commitments to psychiatric research, development, and training; and by holding out as acceptable a less than adequate care delivery system. Denber believed the recession of the 60s produced a concern on the part of state governments as to their ability to continue to fund psychiatric hospitals and clinics. Manpower shortages eroded the capabilities of these facilities and increased the public pressure upon them to release patients. At the same time, the Veterans' Administration system enlarged its psychiatric operations, which produced an acute shortfall of psychiatrists to staff its facilities. These changes collectively permitted clinical psychologists to move into the breach, where they became responsible for the delivery of many psychiatric services. Denber saw the role of psychiatrists within these systems as one of little more than providing medical-legal coverage for the other disciplines. "Psychotherapy at this time became the goal and province of psychologists, social workers, counselors, ministers, and all others who so desired." (Denber, 1978)

Psychiatry continued to take a back seat to the new team concept and cloaked itself in nondirectiveness while preserving the "dignity" of the other team members. In so doing, it relegated its accountability to the patient and took on the role of the hospital superintendent in "One Flew Over the Cuckoo's Nest," a role of benevolent ineptitude.

Ludwig summarized our plight when he said that psychiatry had become a "hodgepodge of unscientific opinion, of sordid philosophy and schools of thought, mixed metaphores, role diffusion, propaganda, politicking for mental health and other esoteric goals (Denber, 1978)."

During this changing period of the 60s and early 70s, the "new therapies" such as tickling and screaming rapidly gained acceptance. Only a fraction of the time and budget that should have been allocated by the Federal Government for the study of neurochemistry, behavioral biochemistry, and psychopharmacology was granted. American graduates of psychiatric residency programs declined from 3300 in 1972 to 2900 in 1975, a drop of more than 12%. At the same time, state and county mental hospitals employed ever-increasing numbers of foreign graduates, until they made up more than 54% of the full-time staffs of these institutions. More than 60% of all psychiatric residents in America in 1975 were foreign-trained. The passage of Public Law 94486 provided support for the training of primary care physicians and defined psychiatric input as necessary in such training programs. Psychiatry initially applauded these "progressive" laws. However, the final effect of this legislation was simply to reduce support for the training of psychiatrists. Public Law 9463, which required an increase in the number of services offered by community mental health centers and increased the numbers of such centers throughout the country, was then passed. Its passage was also widely acclaimed by psychiatry, since the NIMH Five Year Plan provided for the development of more than 860 new mental health centers by 1981. However, the role of psychiatry in these centers and maintenance funding for psychiatric physicians has steadily declined. In fact, the mean number of psychiatrists employed in community mental health centers has declined dramatically — in 1975, only 4.6% of the staff of such centers were psychiatrists. During the past 12 years, the number of psychiatrists administrating such centers has been reduced by 50% while other mental health disciplines have assumed increasingly powerful leadership roles that have permitted them to determine the direction of patient care. Once in positions of leadership as administrators or directs of these centers, psychologists and social workers were, in many cases, able to employ general practice physicians to meet the medical requirements of the centers and thereby insure their own power.

Since 1969, federal support for psychiatric training has diminished by more than 64% in real dollars. The national Institute of Mental Health spends only 30% of its monies on psychiatry. Since the role of psychiatry has already been significantly reduced, current legislative proposals supported by the American Psychological and other nonmedical therapy associations suggest that monies for psychiatry be curtailed even further and used to support paraprofessional training programs. The political thrust has thus been to weaken the position of psychiatric medicine under a guise of functional egalitarianism and better patient care.

During this time, as the public outcries of psychiatric abuse were heard, federal and state governments began to impose more regulations to control psychiatry. Second opinions were required in some jurisdictions for ECT, psychiatric review boards sprung up, and citizen's control groups were increasingly mandated by funding legislation. Our own cry for a holistic model was used to suggest that the psychiatrist should be only a small part of the patient care team. We were now part of the health care "industry" and, as such, became increasingly subject to government regulation and control by "contract law." We had come full circle. The confusion of this position was quite clear, for as Denber (1978) points out, "Changing words and adding phrases did not cure the patient." We needed to face the fact that if psychiatry were a medical specialty, there could be only one model for its practice, "the medical model." To further quote Denber (1978), "Psychiatry is rapidly losing the right to speak for the patient, for psychiatry, or for medicine in general. It also loses the right to consider itself a specialty among other medical specialties."

TERMINAL OR HEALING?

After all of this, where do we stand? Torrey (1978), of the National Institutes of Health, suggests that psychiatry is obsolete as a speciality and will shortly go out of existence because of a lack of patients. He sees the social model upon which psychiatry has been built as the instrument of its demise, since individuals with problems of living will be seen to be in need of educational assistance rather than medical care paid for by the government, while the major psychiatric disorders will soon yield to biological interventions and treatments administered by physicians of other specialties. Torrey suggests that current psychotherapy research demonstrates that psychiatric activities are purely educational in nature and have nothing whatsoever to do with the field of medicine. He believes that people with "brain disease" will be treated by internists or neurologists, while people with problems of living will happily become educated about themselves by seeing psychologists and social workers. Psychiatry will be left bereft of patients, and without patients, it cannot exist. Its future as a medical specialty is nonexistent. To invest in it for the future would be to invest in the Erie Canal as an important future transportation system. Psychiatry is not a growth stock, rather, it will shortly be removed from the big board altogether."

West (1978), eternally optimistic, suggests that psychiatry should work toward overcoming its own internal apathy and strife, and redevote its energies to substantiating its medical identity by developing closer ties with the rest of medicine. In addition, he suggests that psychiatry would be well served if it begins to (1) provide more relevent material to the public, (2) increase the amount of time its skilled members have with the media, (3) develop better and more interesting educational programs for general physicians, (4) enhance its self-evaluation, and (5) exert a greater leadership role in social and political arenas where crucial mental health decisions are being made.

Jerome Frank (1977), long a prophetic voice in our midst, sees psychiatry as a healthy invalid that will recover and continue to play a dominant role in its traditional domain and an increasingly important role in the study and treatment of medical and surgical illnesses. Frank sees the field as being in a period of transition rather than decline and believes that it is "certainly not morbid." He sees new areas of expertise developing from clinical research directed toward understanding (1) the effects of stress, immunological reactions, and disease; (2) the harmful and beneficial effects of medical and surgical procedures; (3) the psychiatric correlates of certain disease states; (4) the interaction of psychological states with hormones and immune responses and, finally; (5) the relationship of brain function to consciousness. Frank is not only perceptive but, I believe, correct, when he defines psychiatry as the only discipline that sits astride the mind-body boundary. Although this is an uncomfortable position at times, it is ultimately one of great import for further medical research and practice.

I also believe that psychiatry will continue to play an increasingly important role with respect to the medical subspecialties. However, it is dangerous to assume that the political forces that have been unleashed will not have a significant and dangerous impact on the field. The dilemma we face today is not that other disciplines may see what psychiatry does as worthless, but rather that they see it as valuable and, therefore, as an element to be incorporated into their practice. Pediatricians have long claimed that pediatries should be increasingly represented in the ranks of child psychiatry or, conversely, that child psychiatry should be increasingly represented in the practice of pediatrics. The same holds true of internal medicine and family practice, where there is a desire to provide more of the biological treatments for psychiatric patients. Such treatments are effective, well defined, and easily taught. The government is already facilitating the diffusion of these skills from our specialty by legislating increased training in the areas of psychiatry for family and general practitioners.

A COURSE OF ACTION

There are many things that psychiatrists, individually and collectively, can do to arrest the processes of role diffusion and political decay. If successful, psychiatry will pass through its current period of stress stronger and more intact than ever before. If, however, we fail professionally to become involved in maintaining the stature and movement of our profession, Torrey's prophecy of doom may prove correct. The field could be politically weakened to such an extent as to become moribund.

Let us look at some of the specific remedies that may be applied to restore the corpus of American psychiatry (Hall, 1979):

1. A recognition that role diffusion has created severe political, educational, and funding problems for the discipline.
2. An increased emphasis on training medical students and residents in the scientific and medical basis of psychiatry. We have long since passed the point where we need to be apologetic for the "soft nature of our science." Psychiatry can be proud of its accomplishments and teach them specifically.
3. Increased efforts at national meetings and through professional organizations, to keep the practicing psychiatrist fully aware of the political pressures facing the specialty. Psychiatry should speak with a clear and loud voice in public forums where issues of physicians' roles and patient management are concerned. In addition, the continuing education of the practicing psychiatrist in the scientific basis of his discipline is essential if he is to present a picture of competence to his medical colleagues.
4. Greater unity among various factions of the discipline. A strong central administration within the American Psychiatric Association speaking cogently for the group and a reduction of intradisciplinary warfare would help accomplish this end.
5. Strong statements decrying the abuse of the mentally ill, made by individuals of stature, such as the heads of local medical societies, district branches, department chairmen, and the APA leadership. We can no longer sit back while other organizations act as advocates for our patients. Organized psychiatry needs to challenge the lack of funding for state hospitals, the lack of adequate research monies from the federal government, the conversion of wings of state hospitals into prisons, and so on.
6. Strong political opposition to all bureaucratically mandated systems that provide less than adequate treatment for the mentally ill.

7. Massive public education programs concerning the role, strength, and special skills possessed by psychiatrists, particularly those that differentiate them from members of the other mental health disciplines.

8. A new unity in maintaining medical control of the treatment team.

9. A limitation to extravagant claims made by psychiatrists concerning what they are able to do.

10. More public education programs designed to enhance the public's awareness of the current state of the art.

11. An end to support of the concept that psychiatric treatment consists only of a warm heart and an extended hand. The neurosurgeon does not profess egalitarianism in the operating room; psychiatry should not express it in the diagnosis and treatment of the mentally ill. Medical diagnosis and treatment remain the province of the physician.

12. A purposeful re-establishment of psychiatry's ties with organized medicine. Such a program needs to begin during the residency years, when psychiatric residents should be encouraged by their training directors and chairmen to learn physical medicine as well as psychiatry. A resident should be expert in the areas of psychopharmacology, somatopsychic disorders, physical diagnosis, medical and psychiatric differential diagnosis, and psychiatric treatment. Unfortunately, we have abrogated many of these responsibilities to other disciplines and, in so doing, have significantly reduced our ability to help many of our patients.

13. A re-emphasis of the fact that the psychiatrist's role is to care for the ill rather than to educate the well.

14. A professional recommitment to scientifically proved truths and treatment values, and the application of research advances to the treatment of the mentally ill.

In conclusion, psychiatry's role will change: Psychiatry will continue to be an important and healthy discipline if its practitioners remember that the philosophy of premum non nocere applies to one's profession as well as to one's patients.

REFERENCES

Coleman, J.S. *Community Conflicts*. New York: The Free Press, 1957.

Denber, H. Is psychiatry in serious danger of elimination? *Psych. News.* 13:17:22, Sept. 1, 1978.

Eaton, J.S., Jr. and Goldstein, L.S. Psychiatry in crisis. *Am. J. Psychiat.* 134:6:642-645, 1977.

Frank, J.D. Psychiatry. The healthy invalid. *Am. J. Psychiat.* 134:12: 1349-1355, 1977a.

Hall, R.C.W., Faillace, L.A., and Perl, M. Role diffusion and "the death of psychiatry," *Psychiat. Opinion* 16:7:21-23,26, July/Aug. 1979.

Laing, R. and Esterson, A. *Sanity, Madness and the Family*. New York: Basic Books, 1964.

Marmor, G. *Psychiatry News.* 13:20:17-44, Oct. 20, 1979. *Psychiatry News.* 13:14:4, July 21, 1978.

Stone, A.A. Psychiatry: Dead or alive? *Harvard Mag.*, Dec. 1976.

Szasz, T.S. *The Myth of Mental Illness: Foundations of a Theory of Personal Conduct*. New York: Hoeber-Harper, 1961.

Torrey, E.R. *The Death of Psychiatry*. Randor Penn. New York: Chilton Book Co., 1974.

Torrey, E.R. What is the future of psychiatry as a medical speciality? Bleak at best. In Brady and Brodie, H.K.H. (eds.) *Controversy in Psychiatry.* W.B. Saunders, Phildaelphia, 1978, pp. 3-12.

Treffert, D.A. Psychiatry's image said to impair patient access. *Psych. News* 13:14:16, July 21, 1978.

West. L.J. The future of psychiatry is bright. In Brady and Brodie, H.K.H. (eds.) *Controversy in Psychiatry,* Philadelphia: W.B. Saunders, 1978, pp. 28-38.

2

Reflections on the Morality of Psychiatry

Earl E. Shelp

The practice of medicine and the provision of health care has been profoundly influenced by its scientific and humanitarian heritage. By careful observation, classification of symptoms, and intense investigation of cause and effect, the storehouse of scientific knowledge has increased throughout the centuries. Physicians have been progressively empowered by scientific understanding to cure diseases and to relieve human suffering to an extent never before known in human history. The persistent quests to unlock the mysteries and to know the secrets of life and death have been generated by an admirable desire to extend and enhance the human estate. The successful application of this knowledge by physicians has helped to inspire awe and to establish the credibility of the medical profession.

The integrity of the medical profession has been enhanced by its moral activity. Chester Burns (1977) and M.B. Etziony (1973) have shown that the philanthropic root of medicine has been reflected in oaths, codes, and prayers throughout medical history. The image of the physician as a competent practitioner selflessly devoted to the well-being of the patient has been shaped by humanitarian service. Subscription to the highest morality and a love of humanity has been viewed as inseparable from the skillful practice of medicine. The physician traditionally has been motivated to benevolently care for the sick and to serve as a model of moral conduct. As a result, the physician and patient are viewed as bound together as friends in pursuit of a common goal (Entralgo, 1969).

The intimate relationship of morality to contemporary medicine is recognized in the Principles of Medical Ethics adopted by the American Medical Association. The special problems in psychiatric medicine were addressed by the American Psychiatric Association (1973) with the adoption of certain annotations to the standard AMA principles. Further, the necessity of ethics to the practice of psychiatry was explicit in the Declaration of Hawaii adopted by the World Psychiatric Association. The preamble stated, "Conflicting loyalties for physicians in contemporary society, the delicate nature of the therapist-patient relationship, and the possibility of abuses of psychiatric concepts, knowledge and technology in actions contrary to the laws of humanity, all make high ethical standards more necessary than every for those practising the art and science of psychiatry" (Blomquist, 1977).

These modern codes offer guidelines for practice, not absolute rules.

Each appreciates the necessity of individual judgment in the application of these standards. The codes implicitly embrace a dual concern: (1) to provide effective care that respects the dignity of the patient and (2) to maintain the reputation of the profession. One could reasonably question, in the light of these admirable emphases on moral conduct and technical competency, why psychiatry is challenged by individuals within and apart from the profession. The extent and intensity of the challenge is evidenced by a cover story in *Time* (1979) in which psychiatry is likened by some of its critics to "modern alchemy." Psychiatry appears to some to have lost its sense of purpose and direction.

Block and Reddaway (1977) attribute the confusion about psychiatry to its ill-defined boundaries of competence, disagreement about the definition of mental illness, use of the mentally ill as scapegoats for the fears of society, and professional conflicts of loyalty. This assessment may or may not be totally correct. Yet, it is indicative of the scrutiny psychiatry is under. Few would deny that the institution is shaken. Its future appears uncertain. A crisis has erupted and an examination has begun.

To suggest that psychiatry is in crisis is to suggest that a turning point has been reached. Clear thinking and wise decisions are required if the goal of the World Psychiatric Association "to promote health and personal autonomy and growth" (Blomquist, 1977) is to be realized. The upheaval within and about psychiatry may be stimulated by a perception that certain practices are ethically questionable and that their theoretical bases are philosophically troublesome.

This essay is written from the perspective of an outsider, an ethicist who has a major interest in medical-moral issues and medical education. These remarks are not intended to discredit psychiatry, dismiss its achievements, or describe its practitioners as morally bankrupt. Rather, the intention is more limited and constructive. I propose to identify several selected conceptual aspects of psychiatry which embody practical issues that occasion ethical reflection and evaluation. I will address these concerns as they relate to the routine practice of psychiatry with the non-psychotic, voluntary, functional patient. This discussion does not exhaust all of the conceptual issues that are of ethical interest, nor does it completely address every feature of the concepts and issues that are included. These are weaknesses inherent in any general essay of limited length and purpose. The selection of concepts is to some extent arbitrary. Others, perhaps more fruitful, could have been chosen from among the options. Some issues in psychiatry are dramatic (e.g., certain modes of behavior control), others are commonplace (e.g., consent), and some are central to the current discussion (e.g., honesty). I have purposefully chosen conceptual concerns that represent these characteristics.

The purposes and methods of ethics are frequently unknown or misunderstood by persons not schooled in the discipline, especially physicians. This lack of familiarity can cause a discussion of medical matters by an ethicist to be seen as an uninformed and unwelcomed invasion of medical territory. This same lack of awareness may contribute to a failure of physicians to receive the assistance of an ethicist in the resolution of a morally perplexing medical decision. This regretful estrangement of two professions concerned for the good of man is being overcome.

The humanities are more and more a part of the medical school curriculum. Ethicists are increasingly recognized by physicians as colleagues disturbed by common questions and in joint pursuit of a common goal. Medical ethicists are not necessarily adversaries of physicians poised to pronounce ignorant criticisms and judgments of immoral conduct. New bridges between the disciplines of ethics and medicine are being built. A mutual learning process has begun. Both will be enriched, and perhaps humbled, by a constructive dialogue. This essay is offered as a contribution to the conversation. A brief introduction to ethics will be given in an effort to define and clarify the perspective of the moral reflections that follow. The ultimate goal of this essay is to increase an appreciation of the importance of moral conduct to the institutional well-being, if not salvation, of psychiatry.

Ethics

Definitions of ethics are as numerous as the textbooks. Some are general and not very technical, others are specific and precisely worded. Arthur Dyck's presentation is one of the more lucid and instructive. He defined ethics as a "systematic reflection upon human actions, institutions, and character" (Dyck, 1977). Ethical reflection is prescriptive, distinguished from the social sciences, which are more descriptive. Ethics is concerned with what individuals and groups "ought" to do, not simply with what, in fact, they do.

Ethics as a discipline is concerned mainly with the normative question of what is right or wrong, good or bad, virtuous or evil. It is also concerned with the non-normative question of the meaning of these terms and their justification. Thus, a chief goal of ethics is to determine if a rational basis can be established and defended for moral judgments, standards, and rules (Taylor, 1975). Ethicists generally pursue their work utilizing one of two major ethical theories: teleological or deontological. Each theory provides a framework within which the normative question can be assessed and the non-normative question analyzed.

Teleological theories state that the ultimate criterion of moral right or wrong is the nonmoral value which results (e.g., pleasure, happiness, health). Utilitariansim is a famous example. This theory asserts that one ought to always do, among the available options, that which will produce the greatest balance of good or value over evil. The good that ought to be maximized is intrinsically, not instrumentally, valuable. For example, autonomy (self-governance) can be considered an intrinsic value, and a surgical procedure necessary to health can be considered an instrumental value.

Deontological theories (of which legalism is an extreme example) deny that the goodness or badness of an act is determined by its consequences alone. For a deontologist, the concept of duty is more important than the concept of good. Deontological ethics is an ethics of duties, not ends. The right action is determined by an application of one or more rules or principles of conduct derived from religious codes, theories of natural law, or other constructs. Examples of rules and principles frequently cited as universally valid, independent of consequences, are truthfulness, justice, and promise-keeping. A right act, consistent with the applicable standard, may or may not produce a greater balance of good over evil. Fidelity to the standard, not a result, is of primary importance to the deontologist (Frankena, 1973; Beauchamp and Childress, 1979).

It is obvious from these brief remarks that ethics is not an exact science. Numerous interpretations or classes of each general ethical theory exist. At times, a deontologist and teleologist may agree, but for different reasons, that a particular act is a right one. On another occasion, for a different circumstance, they may part company. Each may offer morally persuasive arguments for two different courses of action. Unanimity does not always result from ethical analysis. This fact is amply demonstrated by the moral disagreement that exists concering certain medical practices, e.g., abortion.

The morality of psychiatry could be assessed from either of these theoretical stances. The theoretical posture that is adopted will tend to prejudice the analysis toward certain conclusions. For example, a teleologist would pay less attention to specific acts and focus more on the ends produced. Certain therapeutic techniques, to which a deontologist might object, could be sanctioned if a desired end resulted. One might superficially describe this evaluative process as "the ends justify the means." A deontologist would not necessarily embrace this logic. On the contrary, certain actions would be objectionable, regardless of the result, if they unjustifiably violated applicable moral rules or principles. A deontological approach will be used in this essay.

Discordant conclusions about a moral issue are evidence of the complexity of moral questions and the pluralism of moral intuition. The value of moral reflection is not weakened by a failure always to reach a consensus. Rather, the urgency of the task is made more explicit. The character of the human community depends on what we permit and forbid ourselves to do to one another, either directly or through our institutions.

Psychiatry and Ethics

Human conduct is the raw material of ethics and psychiatry. All forms of human activity are of interest to ethics. However, ethicists are powerless to change behavior except by means of rational persuasion. Psychiatry, on the other hand, is not so impotent. Psychiatry studies more than action itself. Psychiatry studies the antecedents and consequences of behavior considered abnormal and intervenes to alter such behavior (Redlich and Mollica, 1976). In certain cases, psychiatric intervention is considered necessary and beneficial to the patient. Society endorses this intervention as a contribution to social order and individual well-being.

Psychiatry is granted certain privileges by society in recognition of its special knowledge and community service. In exhange, the institution is expected to conduct itself prudentially, certify the competency of its practitioners, affirm the efficacy of its procedures, and discipline its members. Formal codes of conduct represent the profession's intention to meet these expectations of society. Even though psychiatry enjoys a special status, as does every branch of medicine, it is not subject to a different moral standard than society as a whole. Psychiatric ethics should be no different from general ethics, except that psychiatrists assume certain special role-related duties.

The true morality of a profession, or any moral agent, is disclosed more in its daily conduct than in its published statements. Some of these daily activities are based on certain assumptions that are themselves composed of a series of unperceived values and beliefs (Columbia University Task Force on Behavior Control, 1979). As noted above, I propose to examine the morality of psychiatry by an identification and discussion of several psychiatric concepts and practical issues that are of ethical concern.

CONCEPTUAL ISSUES

Theoretical and conceptual foundations are an important resource to an investigation of any field of inquiry or practice of a profession. This is true whether the object of investigation is philosophy or medicine. Psychiatry, as a branch of medicine, shares much of medicine's scientific and humanitarian heritage. Yet, psychiatry can be distinguished from general medicine by its definition of illness and therapeutic techniques.

In this section, I shall examine the scope of psychiatry, which is influenced by its view of illness, the impact of values on numerous therapeutic schools, and the relationship of morality to psychiatry.

Scope of the Profession

One's definition of illness will largely dictate the personal, professional, and social response to its discovery. The concept of health is almost universally recognized as difficult to express concretely and define uniformly. Cultural factors, which vary so widely, are critically important to any particular statement of health. This fact renders an exact definition almost impossible. Illness or disease, on the other hand, has been throught to be subject to a more precise understanding, though it too is influenced by cultural factors. Three broad categories, or models, of disease have been suggested.

The first is a somatic model, which holds that disease is a process of inflammation or degeneration of tissue, which may lead to further change or death. The second model is mathematical. Disease is a significant statistical deviation from an alleged norm. The third model is functional. Disease is understood as an inability to function in society. Psychiatry appears to adopt the third model (Hellegers, 1977). Consequently, people who present behavioral and mental symptoms, considered abnormal, as opposed to organic symptoms, are thought to be mentally ill and subject to psychiatric intervention.

In the nineteenth century, a person was considered crazy or insane if he was totally irrational and his behavior was consistently bizarre. These characteristics were easily differentiated by most people from "normal" behavior. However, the definition of madness or mental illness has been less "simple" since the Freudian revolution in psychodynamics. In the post-Freudian era, the definition of mental illness has expanded, its diagnosis has grown more sophisticated, and the scope of psychiatric authority has broadened.

Three stages in this process of expansion can be identified. First, isolated aspects of behavior, rather than the whole personality, could be aberrant but present within an otherwise normal personality (e.g., phobias and compulsions). Next came character disorders. One could be considered mentally ill when a personality trait became a symptom of a constricted character structure not geared toward happiness (e.g., obsessive-compulsive type). Finally, significant behavioral omissions became mental illness. It is normal for certain behaviors to be present. An absence of these behaviors is viewed as abnormal, a sign of neurosis, and therefore, a symptom of mental illness (e.g., desire to die). Thus, less and less became required to define mental illness and more people became classified as deviant or mentally ill (Gaylin, 1976). The territorial boundaries of psychiatry were extended and the influence of the institution increased proportionately.

An "anti-psychiatry" movement has sprung up in reaction to this extension of the illness lable. The criticism by Szasz (1963; 1974) is typical and well known. He restricts the concept of illness to physical disorder, claims that "mental illness" is a metaphor for "moral" problems (socially undesirable behavior), and suggests that psychiatry has become a moral and political enterprise, not a medical one.

The hyperbolic criticisms of Szasz are perhaps simplistic and inaccurate. They do, however, signal the potential for the fraud and abuse of psychiatric concepts. Psychiatric theory lacks a firm, absolute, comprehensive foundation. Use of the word "theory" indicates its tentative basis. Models and systems are constructed, in ways much like other scientific disciplines, to provide frameworks within which thought and behavior, rational or irrational, can be explained and understood. Norms are presupposed but are not exceptionless. Diagnoses of obviously severe disorders made within this framework generate little disagreement. Judgments about non-severe, or borderline, cases are more controversial. Here the implicit warning in Szasz' argument merits consideration.

The public has accepted eagerly, in many ways, judgments of the profession as trustworthy. Psychiatric diagnoses and labels have become common currency in everyday conversation. Unfortunately, however, the concepts and labels have been poorly understood and frequently used inappropriately. The ignorance of the lay public has joined with the endorsement of legal sanction to increase the influence and power of the institution beyond reasonable limits. Further, the mystery that surrounds psychiatric assessment serves to equate psychiatric tratment with madness. As a result, psychiatric patients are often stigmatized and subject to public discrimination. One could question, in some cases, if a "cure" is really better than living with the "disease."

A nonspecific label of mental illness is applied to many types and degrees of mental and behavioral malfunctioning. A diagnosis is valuable to the development of a plan of treatment and as a summary of a person's problems. As such, diagnostic labels are appropriately applied to *patterns* of thought and behavior. On the other hand, when they are applied to a *person* they can become disabling, rather than enabling, to social interaction. Public reaction to an assessment of "schizophrenic" is markedly different from that to "hypertensive." The image of hypertension is one of a *person* with a circulatory disease. The mistaken image of a schizophrenic is one of a *nonperson*, a something different from everyone else. Since a schizophrenic is perceived as a different kind of entity, he is to be avoided, not trusted, and a threat to be removed from the social order.

The effect of some psychiatric labels is a depersonalization of the patient. A nonperson is not given the same respect or protection as a person. The care and custody of a nonperson can be more inhumane than that due a person. The inherent dignity of a psychiatric patient who has been transformed into a nonperson by a diagnostic label may be ignorned or unrecognized. Serious mistreatments by the public, and possibly by the profession, may ensue in disregard of the ethical principle of respect for persons. The rule of reciprocity cautions against an indiscriminate violation of this principle. The counsel of the Golden Rule (Do unto others as you would have them do unto you) provides material content to the standard of respect for persons. The power of psychiatric labels to distort moral rights and obligations required their judicious use and interpretation whether the consultation is voluntary or involuntary.

The legal recognition of and response to psychiatric labels has served to increase their power. A judgment of mental illness may have serious legal and moral implications. The freedom and autonomy of a person are at risk in civil cases. Punishment or treatment are at stake in criminal procedures. A judgment of mental illness can lead to an involuntary commitment to a mental institution in order to protect society, or to protect the patient, or to provide therapy for those unable to make their own decisions. A judgment of mental illness can redirect the management of one's affairs to a guardian or conservator. A judgment of mental illness can relieve an accused person from standing trial or can lead to a verdict of not guilty by reason of insanity (Kittrie, 1978). The benevolent intention of psychiatric involvement in the legal context is virtuous. However, the potential for injustice as a result of the legal enforcement of an inaccurate psychiatric judgment warns against the careless association of psychiatry with law.

The theoretical nature of psychiatry and the imprecise character of psychiatric diagnosis has been vividly demonstrated in the legal context. The cases are legion in which the expert testimony of respected, competent, reputable psychiatrists has been at opposite ends of the spectrum. The credibility of the profession is strained in these instances. The public has grown to expect, reasonably or not, precision and consistency in medical diagnoses. They assume that all medical diagnoses are issued on the basis of scientific fact. Diagnoses made on the basis of impressions and observations frequently are not understood, at best, and rejected, at worst.

Psychiatry is practiced at the pleasure of the state and the people. The profession, as a part of the medical establishment, is presumed to serve primarily the best interests of the patient. The profession also has been called upon to assist the state in the administration of justice. A delicate balancing of interests is required in the legal arena if the integrity of the profession is to be preserved. Entangling alliances may increase the power of psychiatry but they may also compromise its credibility. Psychiatry can suffer, as did the Church, from a too cozy relationship to the state and its interest.

In light of the general presumption of interests, clear and complete disclosure to the client and public of *additional* interests is incumbent on the psychiatrist. A failure to inform constitutes deception and tends to violate the ethical rule of veracity (truth telling). The right to self-defense has been long recognized in ethics and law. This right can be unjustly overridden at the expense of the client by psychiatric testimony given on the basis of information deceptively obtained. To advise disclosure is not to deny that cases may exist in which the interests of other parties are paramount. To advise disclosure is to affirm that the burden of justification for deception rests on those who advocate it.

The legal response to a mental illness label can involve a restriction of personal liberty. The heightened ability of the state to effectively limit the freedom of an individual against his will, as opposed to the less effective means of social disapproval, calls for a circumspect involvement of psychiatry with the courts. When psychiatric involvement is warranted, the testimony must not misrepresent or gloss over the limitations of psychiatric theory, diagnosis, and therapy.

The courtroom can provide a forum for public education. People tend to be afraid of concepts and entities they don't understand. These unknown or poorly understood things can be seen as threats that ought to be removed. This logic may describe the attitude of many people toward those who carry a psychiatric label. The mentally ill patient becomes an unknown entity to a fearful public that has been incorrectly schooled to think that the only way to treat the illness is to remove it (i.e., the person) from society. Perhaps the dark clouds of mystery and misinformation that popularly surround mental institutions and psychiatric offices can be lightened by an honest public disclosure of what psychiatry can and cannot do. This stance is indicated by ethical principles and would appear to serve the interests of the profession and society.

The gradual, yet persistent, extension of the concept of mental illness to include less severe "abnormal" behavior has had a profound impact on the nature and boundaries of psychiatry. Problems in living have, in some instances, become illnesses subject to psychiatric intervention and control. Serious illness that is apparent to all provokes little controversy. The validity of borderline, or less severe, diagnostic catagories are more disputed. These grey areas persent a greater opportunity for unethical, or at least questionable, professional conduct. Indeed, legitimate differences of opinion can reasonably exist. The fact of disagreement no more destroys the validity of psychiatry than it does the discipline of ethics. The disagreement does, however, illustrate the need for a conservative use of the labels of deviance or mental illness.

A label of mental illness may benefit or burden an individual. It may serve as an entry to needed, and perhaps desired, help. It may also serve as a vehicle to undue social discrimination and legal injustices. The potential harm to all concerned that can result from the casual use of psychiatric labels may be not only unfortuante, but perhaps also irreversible and destructive. A recognition of the impact of psychiatric labels, which stems from an inclusive concept of mental illness and the resulting expansion of the institutional domain, counsels their deliberate, accurate, and prudent use.

Therapeutic Schools[1]

The disparity of views concerning the proper limits and applications of the concept of mental illness is reflected by the existence of several psychoanalytic and psychotherapeutic theories. An assessment of the relative strengths and weaknesses of each school is beyond my expertise. I assume that each school has merit. As an ethicist, I am more interested in the concept of human nature presupposed by each theory. Further, I am interested in the implicit and explicit values of each. Therapeutic schools can be grouped within three broad categories: individual psychodynamic psychotherapies, behavior modification therapies, and group therapies.

Individual psychodynamic psychotherapies are variations of the classical psychoanalytic theories of Sigmund Freud. The interpersonal or ego therapies of Jung, Adler, Rank, Horney, Sullivan, Fromm, Rapaport, and Erikson; the instinct therapy of Reich and his popular heirs; and the client-centered therapies of Rogers, Maslow, May, Frankl and Laing fall within this category. Although there is much to distinguish each from the other, they share certain characteristics. They share a common therapeutic technique of conversation between therapist and client. They understand behavioral problems in terms of a common personality theory that emphasizes motives and conflicts. They share a common goal of self-understanding and increased behavioral choice. They share the dominant value of individual well-being and autonomy that guides each.

Behavior modification therapies are based on learning theory. Their therapeutic techniques aim to change bothersome behavior that is seen by the client or society as maladaptive or anxiety-producing. Behavioral therapists are more action- than insight-oriented. They seek to alter behavior by gradually removing reinforcement for an unwanted behavior (Wolpe, Stampfl, Eysenck, Lazarus); or they seek to form new behavior by selective positive reinforcement (Skinner, Bandura, Rotter). The techniques are presented as value-neutral. Only implicitly are value questions addressed when the behavior to be altered is labeled undesirable and when the goal of treatment is specified. The ultimate aim is to permit more consistent functioning, not necessarily increased choices.

---

[1] I have relied on the work of W.M. Sullivan (1978), R. Macklin (1973) and C.J. Rowe (1970) for the categorical and descriptive materials in in this section.

The general category of group therapies represents a variety of therapeutic systems: growth-encounter groups, family groups, milieu therapy, and so on. The radical or sociopolitical therapies of Rogers, Peris, and Berne accept the goal of self-knowledge and aim to enable the client to accept a pluralism of purposes within a social setting. The "new group therapy" of Mowrer advances the idea that anxiety is removed by an acceptance of the violated norms that produced it. Both classes of therapy substitute, as the therapeutic vehicle, social interaction for the client-therapist relationship. Each responds to existing social values: the radical therapies promote democratic change; new group therapy promotes the conservation of existing values and institutions.

Sullivan (1978) suggested that three basic models of human nature underlie and inform the therapeutic schools. The biological-functional model views man as (1) a self-assertive organism capable of modification but not changed by learning or the environment (Freud, Reich); or (2) an adaptive organism capable of fundamental change in response to the environment (Wolpe, Skinner). The intentional-phenomenological model views man as projecting symbolic meaning onto experience. Two variants exist: (1) the individual is more or less free of social constraints capable of creating personal meaning and commitment (Frank, Maslow, early Rogers); and (2) personal meaning is based upon shared cultural symbols and identification with others (Alder, Sullivan, Horney, Fromm). The social-interactional model places the individual within the stream of human interaction that affects behavior. The norms that guide human conduct evolve from the interaction and the environment. One subtype of the third model values creativity and individual expression within the stream of interaction (Fromm, Alder, Reich). A second subtype stresses the control by environmental factors, which requires mutual adjustment.

The foregoing analysis is sufficient to demonstrate the close relationship of therapeutic schools to theories of man. The value-laden character of the respective schools and their corresponding philosophical anthropologies is apparent. Each theory or model of man provides an image of ideal man and an explanation of his deficiency. Consequently, each school has developed therapeutic techniques consistent with the chosen theory to assist man to become what he ought to be.

Characterizations of the human personality that are less than the ideal type are descriptive *and* normative statements. They express negative value judgments when the described individual deviates from the ideal. The correspondence of these jusgments to social values can be explicit (group therapies) or implicit (individual psychodynamic psychotherapies and behavior modification therapies). There is no such thing as value-free therapy. The ethical rule of veracity requires the disclosure of the value commitments inherent in the therapeutic context. Every psychotherapeutic encounter involves the value systems of the patient, the therapist, and the theory. The relative weight given to each of these systems will influence the goal and outcome of therapy. An identification of these values would serve the informed character of the client's consent to participate in the therapy. It would also enhance the client's ability to assume control of his life.

Deception in the therapeutic context can be destructive rather than constructive for the client. It may result in misinformation that obscures a reasonable objective. It may eliminate or obscure relevant alternatives of actions. It may increase uncertainty when the relevant facts are not made known. Instead of the patient being advantaged by the deception, albeit for stated benevolent purposes, he may be disadvantaged (Bok, 1979). Upon learning of the deception, the client may lose trust in the integrity of the therapist and/or the credibility of the therapy. A double standard often exists in a therapeutic relationship: Absolute honesty is required of the client and deception by the therapist is allowed. The counsel of Freud concerning the effect of this unequal standard on the profession is perceptive. Freud wrote, "since we demand strict truthfulness from our patients, we jeopardize our whole authority if we let ourselves be caught by them in a departure from the truth" (Freud, 1979, p. 233). The best way not to be caught is not to commit the offense.

The lure of paternalism (interference with a person's liberty of action for his own good) can be strongly attractive in psychotherapy. An invocation of the "patient's best interests" can cover a multitude of sins. The underlying theme of these remarks has been that the most ethically defensible goal of psychotherapy is restored individual autonomy (capable of making and acting on rational decisions). This is not to suggest that all interventions for a person's own good are improper. At times, restrictions of liberty can be virtuous acts in respect of persons. Gerald Dworkin's analysis of this issue is insightful. Dworkin (1972) suggested that the intervention of choice is the least restrictive alternative and of the shortest duration to reach the desired end. Three types of acts may permit intervention: (1) circumstances in which a proposed act is not in accord with one's actual preferences and desires (psychotic, hallucinogenic drugs) or is destructive and irreversible (addictive drugs, suicide); (2) situations of extreme pressure, which distorts rational perception (challenge to prove courage by dueling); and (3) instances in which a person's decision involves unrecognized dangers to himself. All three instances are extreme, unusual situations of nonautonomous action. Deception and/or restraint may be indicated. The intervention takes place in order to restore the possibility of autonomous action. Otherwise, deception does not appear to serve the interests of the client, profession, or society.

An identification of the values operative in psychotherapy respects the client as a free agent who presumably can participate in the assessment of his best interests. Disclosure helps to guard against the therapist unwittingly becoming a "secular priest" dispensing and imposing his or society's values on the client (London, 1964).

The impact of values on psychotherapy is strong. Social and personal values largely influence what behaviors are considered anxiety producing and abnormal. A behavior so considered is regarded as symptomatic of mental illness subject to voluntary or involuntary treatment (alteration). Thus, the extent and type of permissible intervention into people's lives depends on an understanding of the values matrix. A client may choose to embrace social values and conform to social behaviors or he may not. Unless others would be harmed by his nonconformity, a restraint of his choices appears unwarranted (except in the instances noted earlier). Methods of influence that limit, overtly or covertly, a person's ability to critically choose values and behaviors that do not materially harm others violate the principle of autonomy. Therapeutic methods that support self-esteem, respect human dignity, are honestly presented, and enhance personal autonomy are preferred.

Values in psychotherapeutic theory and practice are inevitable and not necessarily bad. Values are an important ingredient to moral life and social order. They influence every aspect of human life. They ought to be identified and clarified. A denial of their existence in and influence on the several therapeutic schools weakens their credibility and distorts their purposes. An admission of the role of values would not necessarily weaken the validity of the therory or the effectiveness of the therapeutic methods. The ethical practice of psychotherapy tends to

require a full discussion of the therapeutic agenda, including the respective operative values, in order to protect the client's freedom.

Psychiatry and Morality

The influence of social values upon psychiatric theory and practice is evidenced additionally by the close association of psychiatry with morality. The term morality is used in this context to refer to conformity to acceptable ideas and conformity to ideal of right human conduct. I am not concerned with discussing the legal enforcement of moral judgments in this section. I indirectly commented on this matter earlier. I am more interested at this point in discussing the nonlegal enforcement of morality, which can be an equally effective means of social control. I want to focus particularly on psychiatry's role in this process.

The institution of psychiatry is not so much a creator and shaper of social values and behaviors as it is a reflector and enforcer. Psychiatrists, individually and as a group, may embrace and advocate many moral standards. This is particularly true for psychiatry in a pluralistic American society as opposed to a more monistic Soviet society. A diversity of values and therapuetic goals are tolerated as long as they fall within the broad framework of Americana. Society would not permit psychiatry to function if, as an institution, it advocated values and behaviors outside of this framework that threatened social stability. These broad constraints do not in and of themselves pose unreasonable limitations on the institution. They reflect a political and professional fact of life. They also reflect the reality that society as a whole has a stake in what its members value and how they live. Psychiatry necessarily operates within these constraints and with this knowledge. As an institution, it is expected to facilitate the efficient and productive functioning of the society and its members.

Psychiatry has been called upon to place its medical imprimatur on changed social beliefs. Certain behaviors once believed to be sinful or criminal are now understood as symptoms of illness for which the agent is not responsible. Karl Menninger (1973) called attention to the role of psychiatry in this process in a book with the poignant title *Whatever Became of Sin?* Menninger suggested that physical, economic, and ecclesiastical punishment is no longer viewed as an appropriate response to certain behaviors formerly viewed as sinful or criminal. Instead of these traditional responses to transgressions, society, aided by the advice and counsel of psychiatry, has negated the violation by reclassifying it and judging the offender as not responsible. Psychiatry and its related disciplines subtly became psychological and spiritual jurists with power to transform sin and crime into symptoms of illness. Instead of viewing certain behaviors as indications for traditional punishments, certain behaviors are now viewed as indications for treatment (an enlightened form of punishment?).

In addition, certain behaviors once believed by the public and endorsed by the profession to be pathological are now understood as simply atypical. The most remarkable example of this shift of public belief and professional sanction was the declassification of homosexuality as an aberrant sexual behavior. Alcoholism, masturbation, suicide and perhaps marijuana use may be additional examples. An increased toleration, sensitivity, and appreciation of diversity can be generally affirmed from an ethical point of view. Yet, an ethical endorsement of this type of shift does not necessarily entail an endorsement of ethical relativity or moral anarchy. A basic commitment to morality continues to serve as a prerequisite for a behavior to be approved. Edward James (1979, p. 252) stated the principle of social toleration as an obligation "to develop a

society which allows for the greatest possible ethical choice and at the same time promote(s) the deepest sense of moral concern." His counsel concerning liberty and social order appears profitable for the moral philosopher and the psychiatrist. Moral and medical confirmation of personal and public policy judgments can help to secure the freedom of those who previously suffered discrimination, harassment, or punishment as a result of an earlier unjust judgment. In these instances, the social role of psychiatry can be liberating and affirming.

Finally, psychiatry has been called upon to lend its authority in support of social judgments of deviance. Gaylin (1974; 1976) illustrates this point in the following way. If a specific behavior is defined as immoral by a religious authority, a person still feels free to accept or reject the judgment and act accordingly without significant public censure. If, however, the same behavior is defined as healthy, and a person is convinced of the truth of the judgment, he will wish to act accordingly. The fear of illness operating under the medical imprimatur is a sufficient coercive force to alter behavior. By redefining morality into medical terms, the nonlegal mechanisms for controlling behavior are expanded and strengthened. By designating certain behaviors as mental illness, psychiatry affirms societal notions of appropriate behavior and warrants the control of persons whose actions are not in conformity with the prevailing social norms (Tancredi et al., 1975). Szasz (1963), with characteristic exaggeration, viewed this practice as "social tranquilization" and dismissed it as an abuse and misapplication of psychiatric prestige and authority.

Once again, Szasz has overstated his case. He and Gaylin, in a less pejorative manner, however, have drawn attention to the potentially uneasy and coercive alliance of psychiatry with morality. Within a professional setting, "normal" is a descriptive term that does not carry a value judgment. Its popular use, however, is not so precise and free of evaluation. "Abnormal" implies "sick," which requires a response of control to the uninformed lay mind. How often is offensive, nuisance, or immoral equated with "sick" by the layman? How great is the temptation for psychiatry to assume the responsibility to treat these behaviors? What role does social conscience play in psychiatry's effort to cure the ills of alocholism, drug addiction, or the problems of the ghetto. I do not raise these questions as implicit indictments. On the contrary, I raise them merely to suggest how gradually and covertly inaccurate public perceptions can distort the strengths of psychiatry and corrupt its purpose.

The proper role of psychiatry via a vis morality is difficult to assess. Two extreme statements set the context of debate. One could adopt the arguments of Lord Patrick Devlin (1975) to justify a psychiatric enforcement of morals. Devlin argued that the morality of the society takes precedence over individual morality. Shared ideas on politics, morals, and ethics are the requisite bonds of society. They are public in nature and essential to social security. As such, individual morality at variance with public morality constitutes a threat to the moral order, which may be controlled in order to preserve society. The collective judgment of the society determines the public morality. It is self-evident. Within this framework society is responsible only for tolerating the maximum individual freedom that does not weaken the integrity of the society.

One could adopt the arguments of John Stuart Mill (1956) to formulate a stance opposite to Devlin. Mill considered restraints a self-evident evil that required justification by those who advocate its use when the conduct is purely self-regarding. This position would value individual conduct at variance with public morality as long as others are not harmed. The threat to society that stems from choice is seen as more supposed than actual. In fact, Mill suggested that the good of society is better served by choice than by conservation of the status quo.

Psychiatry is called upon to mediate these extremes in everyday practice. The balance between social control and patient care is difficult to strike. The respective goods of individual choice and social order each merit affirmation. The covert threat of conflicting agency is again presented. Does the therapist serve the interests of society or the interests of the patient? Is a defense of the public morality a sufficient reason for psychiatry to abdicate its service to the patient in favor of the interests of society? At what point does nonconformity become a genuine threat to public welfare sufficient to merit constraint? How essential is socialization to individual well-being and social welfare? These are perplexing questions that represent profound practical and theoretical issues. They defy easy answers and perhaps rightly so, in light of their importance.

A determination of the legitimate and beneficial social role of psychiatry will require wide and thoughtful discussion. Where the lines of responsibility ultimately are drawn is vitally important to the well-being of all. The character of society, the integrity of the profession, and individual moral freedom hang in the balance.

CONCLUSION

This essay has been an attempt to contribute to the developing dialogue between the disciplines of ethics and psychiatry. I have attempted to be constructive in suggesting that the moral practice of psychiatry is an essential to its welfare as its technical competency. The institution will not enjoy the confidence of the public if its practices and practitioners are viewed as immoral. To prevent this, the profession must guard against immoral conduct as vigorously as it guards against technical incompetency.

I have identified and commented on three conceptual issues that merit careful consideration by the profession if its moral integrity is to be preserved. First, I suggested that the inexact nature of the concept of mental illness can lead to injustices as a result of the misuse and misunderstanding of psychiatric labels. Second, I suggested that the number of therapeutic schools indicates the inexactness of the science of psychiatry and its value-laden nature. Third, I suggested that a too intimate relationship of psychiatry with morality can result in the institution becoming an agent of social control in contrast to an agent of restored individual autonomy.

An essay of this type can do little more than explore concepts, identify disturbing elements, and invite additional research. I have reflected on selected aspects of psychiatry from the disciplinary perspective of ethics. These reflections are not meant to provide an exhaustive critical examination of psychiatric theory or practice. Rather, these comments are meant to illustrate the importance of (1) honesty, and (2) respect for the moral agency of persons to the ethical practice of psychiatry.

REFERENCES

American Psychiatric Association. The principles of medical ethics with annotations especially applicable to psychiatry. *American Journal of Psychiatry* 130:1058-1064, 1973.

Beauchamp, T.L. and Childress, J.F. *Principles of Biomedical Ethics.* New York: Oxford University Press, 1979, pp. 20-55.

Bloch, S. and Reddaway, P. *Psychiatric Terror: How Soviet Psychiatry is Used to Suppress Dissent.* New York: Basic Books, Inc., 1977, p. 23.

Blomquist, C.D.D. From the Oath of Hippocrates to the Declaration of Hawaii. *Ethics in Science and Medicine* 4:139-149, 1977.

Bok, S. *Lying: Moral Choice in Public and Private Life.* New York: Vintage Books, 1979.

Burns, C.R. (ed.). *Legacies in Ethics and Medicine.* New York: Science History Publications, 1977.

Columbia University Task Force on Behavior Modification. The case of José. *Man and Medicine* 4:2, 1979.

Devlin, P. Morals and the Criminal Law. In *Ethics and Public Policy,* T.L. Beauchamp, ed. Englewood Cliffs, N.J.: Prentice-Hall., 1975, pp. 241-252.

Dworkin, G. Paternalism. *The Monist* 56:64-84, 1972.

Dyck, A.J. *On Human Care: An Introduction to Ethics.* Nashville, Tenn.: Abingdon, 1977, pp. 22-23.

Entralgo, P.L. *Doctor and Patient.* New York: McGraw-Hill, 1969.

Etziony, M.B. *The Physicians Creed.* Springfield, Mass.: Charles C. Thomas, 1973.

Frankena, W.K. *Ethics,* 2nd Ed. Englewood Cliffs, N.J.: Prentice-Hall, 1973, pp. 14-17.

Freud, S. Collected Papers, II. In *Lying: Moral Choice in Public and Private Life,* S. Bok (ed.). New York: Vintage Books, 1979.

Gaylin, W. Foreword. In *Moral Problems in Medicine,* S. Gorovitz, et al., eds. Englewood Cliffs, N.J.: Prentice-Hall, 1976, pp. xxi-xxv.

Gaylin, W. On the borders of persuasion: A psychoanalytic look at coercion. *Psychiatry* 37:1-9, 1974.

Hellegers, A. Round Table Discussion. *Philosophical Medical Ethics: Its Nature and Significance,* S.F. Spicker and H.T. Engelhardt, Jr., eds. Boston: D. Reidel Publishing Co., 1977, pp. 226-227.

James E.W. A Reasoned Ethical Incoherence? *Ethics* 89:240-253, 1979.

Kittrie, N.N. Labeling in Mental Illness: Legal Aspects. *Encyclopedia of Bioethics III:* 1102-1108, 1978.

London, P. *The Modes and Morals of Psychotherapy.* New York: Holt, Rinehart and Winston, 1964.

Macklin, R. Values in psychoanalysis and psychotherapy: A survey and analysis. *American Journal of Psychoanalysis* 33:133-150, 1973.

Menninger, K. *Whatever Became of Sin?* New York: Hawthorn Books, 1973.

Mill, J.S. *On Liberty,* C.V. Shields, ed. Indianapolis, Ind.: Bobbs Merrill, 1956.

Psychiatry on the Couch. *Time,* April 2, 1979, pp. 74-82.

Redlich, F. and Mollica, R.F. Overview: Ethical issues in contemporary psychiatry. *American Journal of Psychiatry* 133:125-136, 1976.

Rowe, C.J. *An Outline of Psychiatry,* 5th ed. Dubuque, Iowa: William C. Brown Co., 1970, pp 4-12.

Sullivan, W.M. Mental Health Therapies. *Encyclopedia of Bioethics III:* 1083-1089. 1978.

Szasz, T.S. *Law, Liberty and Psychiatry: An Inquiry into the Social Uses of Mental Health Practices.* New York: Macmillan, 1963.

Szasz, T.S. *The Myth of Mental Illness.* New York: Harper and Row, 1974.

Tancredi, L.R., Lieb, J., and Slaby, A.E. *Legal Issues in Psychiatric Care.* New York: Harper and Row, 1975, p. 155.

Taylor, P.W. *Principles of Ethics: An Introduction.* Encino, Calif.: Dickenson Publishing Co., 1975, p. 1.

3

The Psychiatrist in the Courtroom: Expert or Advocate?

William W. Taylor, III

Psychiatrists and other mental health professionals[1] are making increasingly frequent appearances in court proceedings. Over the last half century, the adversary system has turned to psychiatry in general and the forensic psychiatrist in particular to help judges and juries decide cases presenting difficult social and moral questions. The most visible, if not the most frequent, of these cases are criminal trials where the insanity defense is raised.[2]

Many court systems have a forensic psychiatric service under the administration of the court, with personnel located physically in the courthouse. Almost any criminal defendant whose counsel requests it can receive an evaluation either by the court's service or by nearby public mental health hospitals. Where a serious question of mental illness arises, the defendant has a right to his own psychiatric expert, to be paid by government funds if he is indigent, and whose opinion is available only to defense counsel unless he testifies.[3] The forensic psychiatrist is now a familiar participant in adversay proceedings and, in the view of many, has substantial impact on their outcome.

---

[1]Including psychologists and mental health social workers, among others.

[2]Psychiatrists also testify routinely in civil commitment proceedings where the issue is whether a person is mentally ill and dangerous to himself or or others; in civil cases, on capacity to make wills or other legal documents, on the extent of mental and emotional damage from private wrongs, and in child custody matters, where the issue is the best interest of the child.

This chapter focuses principally on the role of the forensic psychiatrist in criminal cases, primarily when the insanity defense is raised. Much of what is said, however, relates to psychiatric testimony in civil and administrative proceedings as well.

[3]*United States v Hazel Gaither*, 391 A.2d 1364 (District of Columbia Court of Appeals, 1979).

Except in rare instances, psychiatrists testify as expert witnesses,[4] and their testimony is governed by special rules of evidence. The law accords the expert a special status. Because of training, skill, and experience, the psychiatrist may give opinions or conclusions on relevant matters, presumably beyond the ability of lay people.[5] Because his ability to draw conclusions is greater than that of persons without his qualifications, he is freed from the historical "facts only" rule. His testimoney is limited by requirements of relevance, but he need not rely solely on facts in evidence.[6]

The expert represents a body of scientific knowledge, one in which there is consistency of opinion based upon accepted data and theory.[7] He is expected to remain above the courtroom fray. Although compensated for his time and skill, he has no stake in the outcome of the case. He testifies with an intent to persuade, but without an interest in the fate of the parties. If he performs tests or evaluations out of court, he has no predetermined outcome in mind. He is retained by one side or the other to give his opinion, not to testify favorably to the party who pays him. It is no doubt an overstatement to describe the current relationship between the law and psychiatry as a "crisis," as this book's title might suggest. There is, however, substantial dissatisfaction among lawyers about the forensic psychiatrist's ability, or perhaps willingness, to conform to the traditional model for the expert. Psychiatric opinion often appears to lack consistency. Psychiatrists can frequently be found on both sides of tough cases, especially those with high visibility. This has raised the question of whether the field has the scientific base to permit its members to be treated as experts.

---

[4]In some cases, the psychiatrist may have relevant factual information and presents it like any other witness.

[5]Rule 702 of the Federal Rules of Evidence defines the admissibility of expert testimony as follows:

Rule 702. Testimony by Experts

If scientific, technical, or other specialized knowledge will assist the trier of fact to understand the evidence or to determine a fact in issue, a witness qualified as an expert by knowledge, skill, experience, training or education, may testify thereto in the form of an opinion or otherwise.

Ironically, the law has always permitted lay witnesses to give an opinion about a defendant's sanity if the witness has sufficient firsthand experience with the defendant. "Ladd, Expert Testimonay," 15 Vand. L. Rev. 414, 419 (1952). The psychiatrist gives his opinion on the issue not because he has firsthand experience but because of his special skill.

[6]Experts are also increasingly freed from nonsensical prohibitions against opinions on so-called "ultimate facts" — issues that are outcome-determinative. Rule 704 provides:

Testimony in the form of an opinion or inference otherwise admissible is not objectionable because it embraces an ultimate issue to be decided by the jury.

It is still improper for any witness, lay or expert, to tell the jury in so many words how to decide the case, however. *3 Weinstein's Evidence,* ¶ 704[01].

[7]*3 Weinstein's Evidence,* ¶ 702[01]. Polygraph results have been excluded because they fail to meet these requirements. So has testimony by proffered experts on eyewitness identification.

Second, in some noteworthy instances, individual doctors have eschewed the restraint necessary to compel respect for their objectivity. Some recent examples are illustrative.

In *In re Rosenfeld*, 157 F. Supp. 18 (D.D.C. 1957), for example, a hospital policy decision to include sociopathy as a mental disease produced an over-the-weekend reversal in evaluation of the defendant's eligibility for the insanity defense. In *United States v Gilbert Morgan*, 185 U.S. App. D.C. 373, 569 F.2d 479 (1977), a dissatisfied prosecutor's phone call to the evaluating doctor, detailing the horrendous facts of the offense, produced an amended report unfavorable to the defendant.

Doctors have been willing not only to hold themselves out as experts on issues that, at best, are within the remote periphery of their expertise, but they have also been willing to involve themselves in pretrial "strategy" discussions with attorneys, and out-of-court efforts to achieve a plea bargain.

In the trial of Patty Hearst, for example, Joel Fort, M.D., called as a witness for the government, testified that, in his opinion, Miss Hearst participated in the bank robbery because she feared death or serious bodily harm at the hands of her captors. Over defense objection, the following occurred:

> Question: Dr. Fort, you will recall, I believe, that I asked you Friday whether you had, as a result of the materials you reviewed, persons with whom you spoke in the case, and the physical objects and premises that you considered, were able to form an opinion with respect to whether the defendant participated, in your opinion, in the bank robbery charged because she was in fear of immediate death, or grave and bodily injury by members of the SLA; and you recall there was an objection, which has now been overruled, to that question. What is your answer, sir?
>
> Answer: Yes, I did form such an opinion.
>
> Question: What was your opinion?
>
> Answer: She did not perform the bank robbery because she was in fear of her life. She did it as a voluntary member of the SLA.

Later, Dr. Fort was permitted to testify that he believed Miss Hearst to be lying:

> Question: Doctor, what can you tell us from a psychiatric standpoint with respect to the claim that she fired the gun at Mel's (Sporting Goods Store) almost involuntarily or instantaneously?
>
> Answer: I find it unbelievable.

Dr. Fort admitted, on cross-examination, that he participated with prosecutors in pretrail "strategy" conferences. He also acknowledged that, in the course of his conversations with Miss Hearst's parents, he told them that it was not in Patty's interest to have a public trial and that they should attempt to dispose of the case short of trial, that is by a guilty plea.

The defense had its own problems with the extracurricular behavior of its witnesses. Louis J. West, M.D., a critical defense expert, admitted that his interview with Mr. and Mrs. Hearst had been conducted over dinner in the Hearst's home. Before Patty was captured, but after she was charged, he had written a letter to the Hearsts suggesting that "powerful legal and medical arguments could be mobilized for her defense.[8]

Although these cases may be significant only as aberrations, they illustrate fundamental concerns. Is psychiatry so fickle in its approach to forensic issues that its value to the adversary system should be re-examined? Do psychiatrists have real difficulty in conforming to the level of objectivity demanded of the expert? This chapter examines some of these issues from the lawyer's point of view. It concludes that there is indeed a need for the law to rethink its approach to psychiatry, but that the responsibility for the imperfections is primarily in the legal system's ambivalence to psychiatry, not psychiatry's abuse of principle. It suggests that rigidly enforcing traditional rules and assumptions about experts upon psychiatric testimony is neither productive nor possible, and that the effort should be abandoned. On the other hand, the psychiatric expert must be prepared to engage in a more productive exposition of his opinion than has been the case to this point, and to avoid conduct that, in any expert witness, is unacceptable.

Some courts have suggested that the expert and the lawyer simply speak a different language and that technical misunderstandings are inevitable. In a celebrated series of cases, the United States Court of Appeals for the District of Columbia grappled at length with standards and definitions that would permit psychiatric terminology to be more meaningful for lawyers, judges, and jurors, without controlling legal outcomes.[9] The American Law Institute strove mightily to produce a definition of the insanity defense that was simple and meaningful.[10] Those were efforts to solve mechanical problems, however. Translation is a problem, in some degree, to all expert testimony. It alone does not explain the tension and imperfection in the way lawyers and psychiatrists relate to each other.

---

[8]Dr. West was Chairman of Psychiatry of UCLA Hospitals. Patty Hearst's mother was on the Board of Regents of the University of California. The prosecutor cross-examined Dr. West effectively on this relationship.

[9]*Durham v United States*, 94 U.S. App. D.C. 228, 214 F.2d 862 (1954); *McDonald v United States*, 114 U.S. App. D.C. 120, 312 F.2d 847 (en banc 1962); *Carter v United States*, 102 U.S. App. D.C. 227, 252 F. 2d 608 (1957); *United States v Brawner*, 471 F.2d 969 (1972).

[10]The ALI definition, adopted almost totally in *Brawner v United States*, abandoned the "product" formulation of the relationship between illness and behavior that had been created in *Durham v United States*. It expressed the issue in dual, but clearer, terms of cognition and volition.

There is also, of course, a tension between the healing objectives of the psychiatrist and the law's normative functions. The latter seeks to determine when society can deprive an individual of liberty or other important rights. The former undertakes to diagnose and treat the sick. The psychiatrist must shift gears when asked not about his view of a subject's need for treatment, but rather about the subject's mental condition at a specific time in the past, and its relationship to his conduct.

There is no real reason to conclude that the psychiatrist misunderstands the questions, however, or that his medical orientation makes it impossible for him to answer them. Distinguishing between controllable and uncontrollable behavior is an inquiry most psychiatrists answer every day. Indeed, skill in making that judgment qualifies the witness to testify about it in the first place.

Unfortunately, the law has not been constant in facing the consequences of its need for expert assistance in this area. Although the law has gradually welcomed the psychiatrist's assistance,[11] it has vigorously proclaimed that the expert shall assist, but not overpower, the jury.[12] It looks to the psychiatrist for scientific assistance but pretends that, like traditional experts, the psychiatrist can answer the relevant questions posed *without* in fact recommending how the case should be decided.

Semantic distinctions notwithstanding, the psychiatrist testifies whether, in his opinion, the defendant acted with free will. This is precisely the question that the jury must decide. Whether we like it or not, the psychiatrist advocates a result. He recommends, hopefully upon the basis of all available facts and superior clinical judgment, how the case should be decided. More than with any other expert, the psychiatrist's opinion not only assists the court's inquiry but, if accepted, it concludes it.

The law can do little to make the language in which the psychiatrist testifies any less conclusive. When both sides present experts, the jury will have to accept one or the other. Because the jury's thoughts are unreviewable, we rarely know the factors that guide that decision. We do know, however, that some psychiatrists have more success than others. To be frank, these are experts who have developed skill in testifying. They are articulate, pleasant, and calm people. They weather cross-examination easily, and concede many points to the cross-examiner. They never take positions that cannot be rationally defended and their opinions are generally carefully qualified. They appear to be reasonable people, not zealots, idealogues, or hired guns, and the jury identifies with them.

The jury can feel comfortable that the expert's values closely approximate their own, and the verdict confirms the expert's final moral view of the defendant's responsibility for his conduct.

---

[11] As noted above, the lay witness can still give an opinion about insanity. See footnote 5.

[12] See especially the discussion in *United States v Brawner*, 471 F.2d at 983:

> There is, indeed, irony in a situation under which the *Durham* rule, which was adopted to permit experts to testify in their own terms concerning matters within their domain which the jury should know, resulted in testimony by the experts in terms not their own to reflect unexpressed judgments in a domain that is properly not theirs but the jury's.

Whether a given defendant is responsible for certain conduct is an inquiry that, even for the psychiatrist, has strong philosophical, even moral, components. To the extent that there is professional disagreement as to the point at which impairment, whether organic or functional, affects free will, different psychiatrists may be expected to reach different results on the same facts. It should not be surprising that defense attorneys and prosecutors have identified experts more likely to support their respective positions in any given case.

The court noted in *Brawner* that, under the "product" formulation of *Durham*, experts more often battled over the question of responsibility than over that of impairment. The court adopted the ALI formulation because it felt that it more carefully restricted the expert to medical questions and reduced the probability that he ultimately gave the jury his own moral or philosophical view of the defendant's blameworthiness.

It must be doubted, however, whether the ALI test, or any other, removes the moral and ethical component from the forensic psychiatrist's opinion. Dr. West, under cross-examination in the *Hearst* case, probably put it best:

> The difficulty with psychodynamic explanations after the fact is that it is almost impossible to find situations which cannot somehow be made to fit the theoretical predilections of the observer.

If Dr. West is correct, it may reasonably be asked why the forensic psychiatrist has any claim to expert status, indeed, why psychiatric testimony should be admitted at all. Is the system not encouraging the jury to accept the witnesses called by one side or the other because they appear to offer a better empirical explanation for the jury's own subjective resolution of the issue? Are we not encouraging the jury to avoid its own duty to make moral decisions by trying to convince it that there is a scientific solution?

The witness should expect and be prepared to discuss his philosophical position and the spectrum of philosophical predilections held by all members of his profession. He should not be offended if opposing counsel inquires about the ratio between his testimony in other cases in favor of, and that opposed to, insanity acquittals.

Barring the forensic psychiatrist is obviously not an acceptable solution. Instead of pretending that we can eliminate the impact of the expert's "theoretical predilections" upon his testimony, however, we must make sure the jury understands that they are at work.

A responsible exploration of the expert's philosophical predilections" in the courtroom permits the jury to evaluate the expert's opinion for what it is: a mixture of science, skill, and subjective judgment. The jury can examine whether the expert's predilections are acceptable to the community in the case at hand and, finally, can bring its own predilections to bear in deciding the defendant's fate.

As with any expert, the lawyer should attempt to identify all of the expert's assumptions, not just those that appear purely theoretical. Probably the most important is the doctor's data base.
Some doctors rely almost exclusively upon the psychiatric interview, for example, in determining whether the subject has a disease or defect.
It is not unusual, in the experience of the author, for psychiatrists to ignore background information and testimony from third parties bearing on the question of illness, because he has not personally verified it.

This approach creates a truncated and unrealistic view of the issue. At the least, if the psychiatrist chooses not to rely upon such information,

or to rely only upon such of it as he personally verifies, he should make
that clear in his report and in his testimony.

Second, what version of the offense has the doctor used? He may
get different ones from the police, the defendant, and from third-party
witnesses. Some doctors, in the experience of the author, feel that they
must assume the facts in the police report. If assumptions about other
facts would cause a modification of opinion, or even a willingness to consider it, those assumptions should be specified and the court clearly
of them. If the assumptions are unspoken, serious injustice can
result, because the doctor does not have the lawyer's ability to produce
witnesses and the lawyer cannot know that he needs to do so.

The doctor's report should also identify specific hospital records
upon which he relies; psychological tests, if any, and the person who
administered them, as well as the opinions of other experts that he may
have read or with whom he may have consulted in forming his own. The
rules of evidence permit an expert to base his opinion upon any source
on which he would ordinarily rely, and there is no inference of undue
influence when the witness relies upon other experts. On the contrary,
the witness who refuses to meet with experts, either those with opposite
views or those who share his own, must explain why he did not. If the
expert does not take advantage of the opportunity for such consultations
when offered, he can expect to be rigorously cross-examined on his
failure to do so.

Finally, to what extent did the doctor make a judgment about whether
the subject was malingering, and what role, if any, did that judgment
play in his opinion. It is apparently difficult for psychiatrists to concede that if the subject lied at random during the interview the conclusions
are subject to doubt. Trial lawyers are all familiar with the shudder they
feel when their psychiatric expert proudly announces to the jury that he
believed every word that a sociopathic defendant told him.

It is, of course, important for the doctor to make some assumptions
about the truth of the history he takes from the patient. Evaluating the
defendant's credibility in an ultimate sense is not really his function,
however.[13] Identifying oneself with the truth or falsity of the facts advanced by one side or the other of a lawsuit is not part of the expert's
job. In fact, it diminishes the value of the expert opinion and tends to
demean him in the eyes of the jury. The more experienced forensic psychiatrists readily admit that their opinion depends upon assumptions about
the truth of the information they have received, not only from the subject
but from other sources. At that point it is up to the lawyers to convince
the jury that information upon which the psychiatrist relied should be
accepted or rejected.

Identifying critical assumptions made by the expert helps define for
the jury the impact of subjective factors upon the expert's opinion. The
lawyer and the psychiatrist must engage in a rational dialogue in order
to do this. The psychiatrist must explain himself. He cannot defend his
opinion by reference to his unreviewable twenty years of experience.
At the same time, courts and lawyers must assure that the expert is not
asked questions that call for judgments beyond his capability. This
problem is particularly acute when the issue is competence to stand trial.

---

[13]Even though Dr. Fort and others were apparently pleased to do so
in the Hearst trial.

Competence involves a complex set of considerations. First, does the defendant have an impairment? Second, what abilities are impaired and how seriously? Third, how will the impairment affect the defendant's ability to defend himself? The psychiatrist can help in ansering the first and second questions, but he has little to contribute to the third.

The psychiatrist's expertise extends only to determining whether the defendant is impaired and, if so, the extent to which impairment affects his various cognitive facilities, including memory, vigilence, control, and narrative faculties. It is the court's job to determine which of those faculties is necessary for the defendant to participate in his trial. Competence depends upon the nature of the case and the need for the defendant's participation with his attorneys prior to, and during the trial. It is a functional test, not an absolute one. If the case is simple, the standard for competence is probably lower than if the case is complex. If the defendant must testify, and recall numerous details and reconstruct complex transactions, as is often true in complex fraud cases, even mild aphasia and confabulation could pose insuperable obstacles to his attorney's ability to defend him.

Thus, when a forensic psychiatrist is asked to evaluate a defendant's competence to stand trial, he should endeavor to avoid answering the question in conclusory terms. He can assist most by explaining to the court whether the defendant will be able to perform specific tasks identified by his counsel. In the psychiatrist's interview with the defendant, he should, to the extent possible, determine how stress will affect his ability to function. Particularly with subjects who present symptoms of organic brain syndrome, psychiatrists should examine for lability or catastrophic reactions by attempting to duplicate some of the stress that a vigorous cross-examination by an aggressive prosecutor will create.

It is ironic that, in competence proceedings, psychiatrists have been encouraged to respond in conclusory terms, while in insanity proceedings, the law has strained to prevent intrusion upon the outcome-determining function of the jury. The psychiatrist is a more valuable commentator upon the proper result in insanity defense cases than in competence proceedings, because the former does not require him to make judgments about what a trial will require. The latter is a mixed legal-factual judgment that courts, not doctors, must make.

Responsibility for improving the dialogue between law and psychiatry rests primarily with the legal system. Little is gained by pretending that the psychiatrist can be restricted to a purely scientific opinion if the correct formulation can just be found. It is more productive to admit that the question of criminal responsibility has a substantial subjective element, even for the psychiatrist, and work to identify that element, as well as the psychiatrist's other assumptions, for the jury.

At the same time, the psychiatric expert must accept the same obligation to avoid unacceptable subjective influences, as all experts must. The following are some general guidelines.

No expert should accept compensation in excess of that normally charged for his services. He should have no retainer relationship with a particular law firm, the office of the prosecutor, or the public defender. He should never agree to testify before conducting his evaluation, and he should never accept an employment agreement contingent on his testimony.

For similar reasons, the doctor who evaluates a defendant should have no stake in the consequences of a conviction or acquittal. If at all possible, the evaluating expert should have no relationship to the treating hospital. A doctor in charge of a ward is in a particularly difficult position when asked to evaluate persons charged with violent crimes. A consequence of his testimony may be placement of the defendant on his ward for treatment. Not only would the treating physician likely prefer not to deal with the disruptive patient, but it is virtually impossible to eliminate the physician's concern for his ability to treat other patients who may be affected by the presence of a violent or disruptive one.[14]

It should be self-evident that the psychiatrist should not become involved in out-of-court efforts to settle cases. since such behavior reduces the impact of his legitimate opinion by providing an excellent vehicle from which to launch an attack on his entire testimony. The doctor serves no one by releasing his "humanitarian" impulses in such a venture, least of all the person he is trying to help.

The expert is not part of the team on one side or the other of a lawsuit. There is a difference between consultation on the issues within his expertise and the kind of war games attorneys engage in. The doctor has no business in the latter.

The law does not change overnight, and one can reasonably expect that lawyers and psychiatrists will continue for some time to be moderately disturbed at what they do to and for each other in the courtroom. The shibboleths will hopefully gradually dissipate, and a more productive relationship will slowly emerge. The more frank we can be with each other, the more productive our relationship will become.

---

[14]Similarly, in civil commitment procedures, the doctor who wishes to treat a patient is probably the worst consultant to evaluate the need for incarceration.

Psychiatry In Crisis

4

Psychiatry, Civil Rights, and the Mental Patient

Daniel A. Searing

INTRODUCTION

> "You don't have to be a constitutional
> scholar to know that the place is a
> pigpen"[1]

Concern for the civil rights of the mentally ill or mentally retarded
— often expressed as a polarizing tension between freedom versus right-
to-treatment — is an upwelling crisis in psychiatry. Emotions run high
for both the legal and psychiatric professions. Attorneys working in
the area of civil rights for the mentally ill or retarded evidence an unusual commitment to their work. Psychiatric staff, equally dedicated yet
hampered by shortages of money and manpower beyond their control,
feel unjustly attacked. One commentator has predicted that pursuit of
reforms in mental health care without recognition of clinical realities
will "plunge us into a new dark age in the case of the mentally ill (Shwed,
1978)."

The "interface" between law and psychiatry is more volatile than in
similar professional interactions, such as those of law and academia.
Issues such as psychiatric evaluations in a legal setting, expert testimony,
informed consent, judicial review of medical decisions, and right-to-treatment make this volatility inevitable.

Yet this confrontation can be a force for good. Out of this challenge
and struggle should come some very basic decisions, both on (1) whether
constitutional rights that *we* as educated, knowledgeable professionals
take for granted are extended to those less able to assert them and
(2) where and how required treatment or habilitation in the least restrictive environment can be best obtained.

Change is facilitated by understanding. In this chapter I wish to
briefly explore the concept of right-to-treatment from an attorney's perspective: a little law, a little political science, a look at where we are
today, and some practical considerations. This may help to smooth the
interface with respect to this one critical issue.

---

[1]Comment of federal judge following visit to Fernald School in Massachusetts, as reported by Stone (1977).

HISTORY AND DEVELOPMENT OF THE
RIGHT TO TREATMENT

The definitive history of the development of the right-to-treatment concept has not yet been written. At this point in time it may not be possible to set it down. There is too much change, too much uncertainty, too much development of both theory and practice. Yet, there is a pattern to the development of legal concepts such as right to treatment. These perimeters on social or professional conduct do not suddenly appear as a revelation. They can even be anticipated — perhaps making resort to the courts unnecessary.

Elementary civics teaches that our judicial system is one of the three branches of our government. We learn that this system functions on many levels: state, trial, federal, appellate. The appellate level — the Federal Circuit Courts of Appeal and the United States Supreme Court — serves to protect various interests in our society, and indeed often fills a vacuum created by the inaction, ignorance, or selfish interests that sometimes exist in our system.

A few examples will illustrate. In commerce, it became apparent that the individual states were going to make a mockery of our federal union by imposing a variety of restrictions on the free flow of goods. During the early part of this century the appellate federal courts were kept very busy striking down these impertinences under the Commerce Clause (*Baldwin v Seelig*, 1935). In the two decades prior to the 1954 school desegregation decision (*Brown v Board of Education*, 1954) the N.A.A.C.P. was carefully orchestrating a series of decisions such that the logical outcome was Brown. In the area of criminal law, egregious police practices presented to the Court led to sweeping changes in search and seizure, warnings concerning arrest, and right to counsel (*Wolf v Colorado*, 1949; *Miranda v Arizona*, 1966; *Gideon v Wainwright*, 1963).

This concept of judicial intervention may be easier to visualize if we imagine the development of the law as a pendulum swinging between sharply competing interests, trying to find the proper balance for issues such as state regulations versus free commerce, equal educational opportunity versus the cultural and social morals of an entire region of our country, the rights of the accused versus the protection of society, and the rights of the committed versus the responsibilities and resources of society.

Much of the movement of the pendulum one way or another is caused by the recognition of a gap between the constitutional standards for the treatment of certain individuals and classes and how society actually treats them. Minority children were being denied the educational opportunities provided whites. Police practices in some cases resulted in the accused being treated as if convicted. The mentally ill were being warehoused and bypassed in terms of the allocation of society's resources. A brief review of some of the factual settings faced by the courts concerning treatment of the impovished mentally ill will illustrate that the disparity of treatment for this latter class of citizen had truly become disproportionate.

Although each factual situation is different, typically there exists in state mental hospitals:
  - inadequate physical structures — old, unsafe buildings, open sleeping areas, barren, poorly lit day rooms, open unsanitary baths, no adequate programming areas. No aspects of the environment meet minimally acceptable standards.
  - an environment that leads to regression, psychological and physical injuries, aggressive and other maladaptive behavior, excessive use of tranquilizers, use of physical restraints.

- inadequate and insufficiently trained staff, far below professional standards.
- inadequate, nonexistent, or inappropriate habilitative programs: inactivity, no recreation, waiting lists for programs.
- excessive use of seclusion and time-out procedures.
- deficient medical and health-related activities.
- life-threatening medication and drug practices.
- few if any community-based services.

These conditions prompted a search for a solution, which often led to an exploration of the constitutional standards of basic individual rights.

Sometimes a social need cannot be filled by looking to the Constitution. The Court has rejected, for example, claims that discrimination on the basis of wealth violates the Fourteenth Amendment, or that the Constitution contains a right to housing (*James v Valtierra*, 1971; *Lindsey v Normet*, 1972). We do not yet know if the particular needs of the mentally ill for decent habitation and adequate treatment can be met through a constitutional standard. The court is still out.

Yet, the early right-to-treatment cases, which dated from as early as 1952 and dealt with the civil commitment of sexual psychopaths, laid the basic foundation for the concepts that have matured in the past decade (Stone, 1975). Early commentary by Dr. Morton Birnbaum in 1960 argues on policy grounds that right to treatment represented an avenue to betterment of deteriorating conditions in mental facilities nation-wide (Birnbaum, 1960).

In 1966 the Court of Appeals for the District of Columbia, in considering an individual confined following a verdict of not guilty by reason of insanity, found a right to treatment in D.C. statutes, and alluded to constitutional concerns such as the Eighth Amendment's prohibition of cruel and unusual punishment and the Fourteenth Amendment's right to due process and equal protection. This seminal case is *Rouse v Cameron*, 373 F.2d 451 (D.C. Cir. 1966). In its opinion, the court outlined a three-part guide:

1. Did the hospital make a good-faith effort to cure or improve the patient?
2. Was this effort adequate according to contemporary standards?
3. Was an initial treatment plan established and updated?

While these queries were fair fundamental guidelines, they whetted legal appetites for their testing. The recipe was merely dissatisfied patients and case-by-case trials! Worse yet for the psychiatric profession – the result of a successful challenge was release! But the impact was zero. Stone (1975) states that no one was released, that the American Psychiatric Association took no initiatives in its reaction, and that a leading forensic psychiatrist dismissed right to treatment as "enchanting legal fiction." The pendulum had barely started to move.

Into this arena, *Wyatt v Stickney* (1972,1974), attacking conditions in hospitals run by the Alabama Department of Mental Health, dropped like a bomb. Hoffman and Dunn (1976) characterized *Wyatt* as the statistical approach: It was a class action, to avoid the case-by-case scrutiny of *Rouse*; community standards were replaced by a numerical approach of detailed objective standards for staff-patient ratios and physical plant. While curing some problems, *Watt* led to others: Bureaucratic survival mandated manipulation of patient numbers and budget requests, and there was an assumption of spontaneous adequate treatment once the numbers were right. Hoffman and Dunn (1976) detailed two shortcomings: where was peer review of the therapist and where was flexibility in treatment?

Nevertheless, in retrospect, *Wyatt* caused an explosion in right-to-treatment cases.

A pause is necessary here to briefly focus on the rationale of these early cases. This is an important exploration because the early cases provide the theoretical base upon which later cases and statutes have been built, and they help to explain the Supreme Court's recent ruling on right to treatment, which will be covered below.

Every person's right to liberty is one of the touchstones of our constitutional system. The right of the State to curtail that liberty in certain circumstances is another touchstone. Police power is one example. The State can act in a variety of ways to protect society from dangerous acts of an individual. A criminal can be confined; but under our system this confinement has several due process limitations:

1. A specific offense must have been committed.
2. Confinement is limited to a fixed term.
3. A proceeding containing certain procedural safeguards must come before confinement (right to counsel, for example).

Civil commitment is also a curtailment of liberty, and as such it must also be accomplished through due process:

1. A legitimate state interest must exist.
2. There must be an appropriate proceeding to establish the reasons for commitment.
3. Confinement must end when the reasons end.

The required state interest in such proceedings has traditionally been grounded on a *parens patriae* rationale — a state may act upon another who cannot make a rational choice for himself, who is dangerous to himself or others.

The early right-to-treatment cases rested on two theories growing out of *parens patriae:*

1. The state's reason for confinement was that the person needed treatment; therefore, not to provide treatment violated due process. The state's reason for confinement was negated by its inaction.
2. Because due process standards for civil commitment are less than for deprivations of liberty because of criminal conduct, the state must offer a *quid pro quo* to justify confinement. This *quid pro quo* is adequate treatment. The absence of such treatment thus tainted the due process proceeding, which in turn mandated a remedy when such taint was established.

This was the basis of *Wyatt* and the 5th Circuit opinion in *Donaldson v O'Conner* (1974). This reasoning also caused Chief Justice Burger much trouble when *Donaldson* arrived at the Supreme Court.

Nevertheless, these cases provided precedents for future decisions. Judges faced with similar issues could look to these cases for guidance — or could try to distinguish them and reject their reasoning.

RIGHT TO TREATMENT AND THE SUPREME COURT

Our federal judicial system mandates that new and evolving constitutional challenges to existing practices be heard first in the district courts. They are then heard by the circuit courts of appeal. If the issues are of sufficient importance, or if there is disagreement among the circuit courts, the Supreme Court will hear argument. *O'Conner v Donaldson* was heard and decided by the Supreme Court more than six years ago, in June 1975. This was a highly publicized case that was considered the lead vehicle for Supreme Court certification of the right-to-treatment.

What were the facts? Donaldson was committed in 1957, following proceedings initiated by his father. A Florida county court judge ruled after hearings that Donaldson was suffering from "paranoid schizophrenia." He was committed for "care, maintenance, and treatment" under a state statute since repealed. Donaldson wanted out and made his requests known. Although hospital staff had the power to release him, O'Conner, the hospital superintendent, refused permission many times. At trial O'Conner expressed concern that Donaldson could not function outside the institution, but could not recall his reasoning for that conclusion. Trial testimony showed (1) that Donaldson had never posed a danger to others; (2) that there was no evidence of suicidal or self-injuring tendencies; (3) that he had worked productively for 14 years prior to commitment (he immediately found a job upon release). Additionally, before trial, O'Conner retired and within weeks Donaldson had both his release and a judicial restoration of competency.

Trial also revealed that Donaldson's attempts at release had been supported by a number of persons who were willing to provide responsible care. O'Conner rejected these offers, stating Donaldson could only be released to his parents – an impossibility since he was 55 at the time. His "treatment" was enforced custodial care. There was some evidence that Donaldson refused medication on Christian Science doctrine grounds. Donaldson's requests for ground privileges, occupational training, and an opportunity to plead his case with O'Conner were denied.

A jury found for Donaldson, awarded damages, and the 5th Circuit Court of Appeals affirmed (Donaldson v O'Conner, 1974).

Now we must pause here to consider two items. First, law suits turn on facts, and the way the facts are presented often provides a clue to a court's thinking as well as determining the result. My distinct impression in reviewing the facts as presented by Mr. Justice Stewart, very much as I have summarized them here, is that the Court had grave question that the case wasn't a one-on-one altercation between the superintendent and the patient. This is not the stuff upon which serious constitutional questions are decided.

Second, in most cases the Court will do anything to avoid a decision on constitutional grounds. If there are procedural problems such as standing (the right to be in court) or case or controversy (is this a real dispute?), or if there is an applicable statute, constitutional grounds will be avoided. I believe this is especially so when the Court is asked to create (or discover) a new right founded in the Constitution.

With this in mind, what was the result in Donaldson? Well, for civil rights lawyers it was a disappointment. Right to treatment was ignored. Worse, in Burger's concurring opinion, the broad-based 5th Circuit opinion conferring a right to treatment was swept aside as precedent. Although this was what lawyers call dicta, these opinions reverberate through the legal system as lower court judges attempt to apply what the Court actually said, what the judges think it said, and what they would believe it said.

For psychiatrists it means that right-to-treatment issues are still going to be fought out in the lower courts, until the appropriate fact situation is brought to the Supreme Court. But the opinion offers guidelines on a narrow, but important, question. The court termed this "every man's constitutional right to liberty." These guidelines are:

1. A state law authorizing confinement of a harmless mentally ill person is not enough to override the right to liberty.
2. Even if the original finding was valid, once that finding changed, right to liberty takes over.
3. A finding of "mental illness" alone is not enough if a person is harmless and can live safely in freedom.

4. Providing a higher standard of living is not a sufficient rationale.
5. Neither public intolerance nor animosity is sufficient rationale.
In the words of the majority:

> "A state cannot constitutionally confine without more a
> nondangerous individual who is capable of surviving
> safely in freedom by himself or with the help of willing
> and responsible family members or friends."

If you feel that, after digesting that homily, we are not out of the briar patch, this author agrees.

As previously noted, Chief Justice Burger's concurrence raises some warning flags for future cases. His role as court spokesman in these cases ensures that the arguments he advances will be made persuasively when the Court again considers right to treatment.

His initial comments were parenthetical to the main issue — but important to professional staff making individualized decisions. Donaldson had petitioned *state courts* on several occasions to get out, and was refused. Whatever the reasons for the refusal and regardless of whether they were right, the hospital staff had grounds for treating each refusal as approval of continued confinement. Such judicial decisions may confer immunity if that same person brings a right-to-treatment claim in federal court.

In commenting on the theories relied on by the 5th Circuit, Burger plainly doesn't buy the right-to-treatment analysis. He agrees that the state must adequately justify confinement and recognizes *need for treatment* as a justification. But he believes a conclusion that a state cannot confine the nondangerous mentally ill except for purposes of treatment is too broad.

First, this is not the way states have operated, so there is no historical justification. Second, the fact that some limits on *parens patriae* power exist should not mean that, with regard to the mentally ill, it can be exercised only if treatment is available. Much mental illness is not understood and many persons are "untreatable" in that there is no therapy. Effective therapy is very difficult without acknowledgment; many mentally ill persons will not acknowledge illness. Others may not be able to function "outside" and may harm themselves. Burger argues that the state legislatures should provide this framework, not the courts.

Burger saves his real scorn for the *quid pro quo* theory — that curtailment of liberty without the many safeguards of the criminal court demands, as a tradeoff, treatment. This theory fails because the safeguards are often tailored to individual cases. Close appraisal of decisions of society to confine some of its members does not mean judges can impose their own "notions of public policy," and that what is basically a concern for procedure is elevated to a new constitutional right. State benefits of treatment are traded for confinement. Burger obviously feels this is dnagerous ground, and I think, on this argument, he is correct. It remains to be seen whether these concerns will be persuasive with four other justices.

While no other cases involving the right-to-treatment issue have either reached or been accepted by the Supreme Court, the Court continues to hear challenges to a related issue, confinement of the mentally ill. The 1978 term produced two cases challenging the procedures by which two states, Georgia and Pennsylvania, handled voluntary commitment of children to state mental hospitals (*Parham v J.L. et. al.*, 1979). Chief Justice Burger, writing for the majority in both opinions, held that the procedures of both states passed constitutional muster in terms of due process.

LEGAL THEORIES: PROSECUTION AND DEFENSE

While right to treatment remains quiescent at the Supreme Court level, there is no question that additional challenges are continually being raised at the lower court level. A variety of legal theories are being advanced, some of which flank Chief Justice Burger's analytical problems. These theories include:

1. *There exists a constitutional right to treatment.* The basic "right to liberty" analysis for this theory has already been discussed.

2. *There exists a constitutional right to be free from harm.* This theory was discussed in *Nyarc and Parisi v Rockefeller* (1973). The court held that a right to be free from harm, to be protected from injury by hospital authorities, is a basic right of a person who is confined. Further, this protection from harm should be the constitutional basis for improved conditions, rather than a right to treatment or habilitation.

3. *There exists a constitutional right to receive habilitative care in that setting least restrictive of personal libery.* Recognizing the state's interest in meeting the needs of its neglected, mentally retarded, or emotionally disturbed persons, this means that treatment least restrictive of personal liberty must be provided. In *Wyatt* the court said this meant a change from
   · more to less structured living
   · larger to smaller facilities
   · larger to smaller living units
   · group to individual residence
   · segregation from to integration in the community
   · dependent to independent living.

4. *Restraints imposed without due process are in violation of the Eighth and Fourteenth Amendments.* This somewhat narrower theory argues that widespread and indiscriminate use of solitary confinement, bed shackles, leather restraints, muffs, and chemical restraints are in reality *punishment,* not treatment to meet constitutional standards; punishment by the state can be imposed only after meeting certain strict due process standards.

5. *There exists a constitutional right to nondiscriminatory habilitation.* In other words, retarded persons have a right to at least as much education and training as the state affords to others. This theory focuses on the Fourteenth Amendment Equal Protection rights of the mentally retarded.

DEFENSES TO RIGHT TO TREATMENT

Most of the previous discussion has focused on the offense. Litigation has two parts, however, offense and defense. Our perspective is sharpened by reviewing some of the defenses that have been advanced.

The basic legal defense is, of course, that there is no right to treatment. The prognosis for this is not good.

Lack of resources is almost always advanced in these cases. There is no question that such a defense is true; bringing the challenged institutions up to professional standards would usually cost many millions of dollars. Unfortunately, truth is only a defense to libel, not to right to treatment. Lack of money has never been a defense to constitutional violations. Justice Blackman once opined the principle: "Humane considerations and constitutional requirements are not, in this day, to be measured or limited by dollar considerations." It is easy to see that this takes away one of the principle defenses in this area. It also should serve to give notice to institutional administrators and state health officers.

"Good faith" is almost always cited as a defense. Again there is usually no question that this exists. It is usually possible to show that tremendous efforts have been made. However, this is not enough to protect a defendant from the constitutional violation. It is, however, very important in another respect. Good faith efforts on the part of named defendants to correct conditions within available resources are enough to protect defendants from personal damages for injuries claimed by plaintiffs. In these situations the courts find against the *institution* and the *system*, rather than the people involved. It is also good law that claims against state officials for equitable relief (meaning that the court orders corrective actions) do not require evidence of malice or bad faith.

Another defense often advanced is the number of improvements made since the start of the original investigation or filing of the complaint. Plans to upgrade or close facilities are held to have little bearing on whether constitutional rights are beging violated *now*.

As to improvements, there is a long line of cases holding that, even where the illegal conduct has ceased, courts will take action unless a defendant can show "there is no reasonable expectation that the wrong will be repeated." This is a tough standard!

The type of relief ordered is an important factor in determining whether to fight a case or settle. Stone, in March of 1977, stated that right-to-treatment cases have precipitated the release of thousands of patients — of course that was the idea. In most cases, however, this is only one part of a highly structured plan.

Typically, the court is asked to immediately enjoin such practices as use of seclusion, brutality, abuse and neglect of patients, the over-use of tranquilizing drugs, feeding patients in supine positions, and the use of physical restraints without adequate monitoring, periodic review, and an individualized treatment plan.

On a somewhat longer term scale, the court is asked to order a survey of individual patient needs and immediate placement in appropriate community-based programs on a priority basis. Often a special master is requested to monitor progress. All of these steps are within the power of the court; none need lead to precipitous discharge.

CURRENT STATUS OF RIGHT TO TREATMENT

Where are we *right now* in right to treatment? The battle is still being waged in the district and circuit courts of appeal. The 1977 favorable decision in *Haldeman v Pennhurst* (1977), concerning a Pennsylvania State School and Hospital, found support in decisions in Illinois (1973), Indiana (1973), Rhode Island (1972), Pennsylvania (1977), Georgia (1976), Louisiana (1976), New York (1976), Hawaii (1976), Alabama (1974), Ohio (1974), Tennessee (1974), Minnesota (1974), Texas (1974), and Wisconsin (1972). The 1st, 2nd, 5th, 7th, and 8th Circuit Courts of Appeal have considered the question, with mixed results. Until one of these cases reaches and is decided by the Supreme Court, right to treatment is still very much an open issue.

SOME PRACTICAL CONSIDERATIONS

This brief overview of but one aspect of the interface between law and psychiatry has attempted to explain some of the development of constitutional theory and the current judicial status of the right to treatment.

Some form of the right to treatment is here to stay. Only the major vehicle for the concept is not yet clear. But whether it be state or federal statute, case law, or professional standards, in closing this chapter some practical considerations provide a good summary.

- Do become acquainted with the state of the law in the jurisdiction in which you are practicing. Have the hospital counsel make an annual presentation. Read the opinions in your state and federal circuits. Read the statutes. They aren't any worse than a psychiatric evaluation or nurse's notes.
- Do take an active part in developing standards for your hospital or unit.
- Do speak out at professional meetings for what you believe are proper standards.
- Don't feel that all lawyers are out to damage the psychiatric profession — it's only a select few, readily identifiable.
- Don't be afraid to challenge statutory provisions or administrative or medical decisions that accomplish or have the effect of curtailing the right to liberty enunciated in *Donaldson*.
- Don't, on the other hand, be afraid to vigorously defend your professional judgment.

ACKNOWLEDGMENTS

Mr. Searing is a Trial Attorney, Civil Rights Division, United States Department of Justice. The opinions expressed herein are solely those of the author and do not reflect the policies of the Department of Justice.

REFERENCES

Baldwin v Seelig. 294, U.S. 511, 1935.
Birnbaum, M. The right to treatment. *Am. Bar. Assoc. J.* 46:499-505, 1960.
Brown v Board of Education. 347, U.S. 483, 1954.
Donaldson v O'Conner. 493 F.2d 507 (5th Cir., 1974).
Gideon v Wainwright. 372 U.S. 335 (1963).
Haldeman v Pennhurst. 446 F. Supp. 1295 (E.D. Pa., 1977).
Hoffman, P and Dunn, R.C. Guaranteeing the right to treatment. *Psychiat. Ann.* 6:6:261-263, 1976.
James v Valtierra. 402 U.S. 137 (1971).
Lindsey v Normet. 405 U.S. 56 (1972).
Miranda v Arizona. 384 U.S. 436 (1966).
Nyarc & Parisi v Rockefeller. 357 F. Supp. 752 (E.D. N.Y., 1973).
O'Conner v Donaldson. 422 U.S. 563 (1975).
Parham v J.L. et al. No. 75-1690, S. Ct. Ga. June 20, 1979.
Rouse v Cameron. 373 F.2d 451 (D.C. Cir., 1966).
Secretary of Public Welfare of Pennsylvania v Institutionalized Juveniles. No. 77 1715, S. Ct., June 20, 1979.
Shwed, H.J. Protecting the rights of the mentally ill. *Am. Bar Assoc. J.* 64:564-567, 1978.
Stone, A.A. Recent mental health litigation: A critical perspective. *Am. J. Psychiat.* 134:3:276, 1977.
Stone, A.A. Overview: The right to treatment — comments on the law and its impact. *Am. J. Psychiat.* 132:11:1126, 1975.
Wolfe v Colorado. 338 U.S. 25 (1949).
Wyatt v Stickney. 344 F. Supp. 387 (M.D. Ala. 1972), aff'd in part 503 F.2d 1305 (5th Cir., 1974).

5

Current Legal Issues Affecting the Practice of Psychiatry

Jonas R. Rappeport

The current emphasis on human rights began in the United States in the early 1950s and has since grown to the point of creating a crisis in some areas of medical practice. While social efforts to better the lot of mankind always swing to and fro like a pendulum, in the current efforts there is still more movement to the "left" to be anticipated, while at the same time there is movement to the "right" to correct excesses. I have previously stated that psychiatry is "belegaled (Rappeport, 1976)." We are caught in a web of regulations, new definitions, due process requirements, reports, and paperwork such as we could not have imagined 30 years ago. Lest we feel paranoid, the new demands have been placed on all professions, even governmental agencies. In our efforts to protect liberty, we may have destroyed some of the forces that motivate people, by "belegaling" ourselves in such a manner as to make it too dangerous to take risks or try unusual or different techniques.

Psychiatry is in crisis and will be for many years, as we search for better solutions to old problems. Two standards of care for the mentally ill, public and private, may be a necessity as in other forms of medical care, but clearly the public sector has needed readjustment. The current solutions, however, may represent excesses in society's attempt to do away with inequities and inequality. Our society's reliance on the judicial system to solve all human problems is destined to failure. This has to be obvious when we look at the mess the judicial system has created for itself without our help. Yet there probably was no other way to correct some of the undesirable aspects of the psychiatric care system. Unfortunately, judicial fiats and clinical judgments are so far apart in philosophical foundations as to make the use of one by the other exceedingly difficult. Yet we must face the fact that we are in an era when professional judgment has been eroded by judicial fiat.

The crisis is not so much the result of suddenly discovering injustices as it is the problems produced by the attempted solution that utilizes techniques that do not lend themselves to solving the problems. The law knows only black and white, allowing little room for gradations when determining whether a commitment law meets constitutional standards, or whether a certain medication may be too risky. Unfortunately, mental illness and medical judgments do not lend themselves to such exactness. Writing notes and reports, making a record of everything, and attending hearings is so time-consuming as to take away from the patient the care he most needs. Unfortunately, we must admit that there were areas in which the care patients received was totally inadequate, if not inhumane. In many cases familiarity made us content with conditions that we should not have tolerated. Now these conditions have been brought to light by the human rights movement. Some have been adequately corrected, but for others the attempted solution has only made conditions worse.

Whether we like it or not, the practice of psychiatry is in a state of change. All areas of practice are affected, as evidenced by the many chapters in this book. Legal issues have affected every facet of our professional lives and the lives of our patients. Before prescribing medication, it is important to be sure we have a fully informed consent or we might be sued. We may need to obtain a second opinion before beginning ECT. We should warn a known third party that his life is endangered. We must seek the least restrictive alternative in our quest for care for our patients. We must watch a potentially suicidal patient as an out-patient because we could not prove, beyond a reasonable doubt, that he was suicidal and in need of in-patient care. These are issues for psychiatry that did not exist 10 years ago, the result of law suits and/or new legislation. A look at some of the areas most affected will reveal the seriousness of the situation.

CONFIDENTIALITY

Psychotherapy, that mainstay of psychiatric practice, has lost some of its security. Patients are willing to expose their innermost secrets only because they believe in the confidentiality of the process, whether it be in an individual or a group setting. Yet, there have been some incursions into this time-honored concept of confidentiality between the doctor and his patient. A recent Supreme Court decision, *Zurcher v Stanford Daily* (1978), allowed a police search of the records of the campus newspsper. This right of the police could be extended to the doctor's medical records when they are searching for evidence regarding a suspected criminal who is in psychiatric treatment (Klein, 1979).

The Tarasoff case has caused extreme concern to psychotherapists, as it has the frightening prospect of raising the responsibility of the therapist to ludicrous levels. In the Tarasoff case, the court stated that a psychotherapist had the responsibility of warning a third party that his/her life was endangered if the therapist believed that there was such a risk (*Tarasoff v Regents of the University of California*, 1976). Tarasoff was a young girl who was murdered by a patient who had indicated to his therapist that he was going to murder her. The therapist attempted to institute commitment proceedings. However, the police did not feel that the individual was so "imminently dangerous" that he required hospitalization, but told him to leave the girl alone. Consequently, the patient became angry at this therapist for having revealed his plan and he stopped treatment. When Miss Tarasoff returned from her vacation, the patient, now not in treatment, murdered her. The court indicated that there was a duty to warn when one in a position of power or responsibility had some reason to believe that a third person's life was in danger. The court pointed out that there were other situations in which such a responsibility existed and that this was only a natural extension of a basically sound social policy. The court stated that psychiatrists had indicated that they had the capacity to predict dangerousness, but now would have one believe that they could not. While this is not the place to discuss the pros and cons of Tarasoff, it was a potentially important decision in that it has placed in fear many therapists whose patients on occasion might threaten violence. While we could generally state that most patients,

particularly those in out-patient treatment, are not particularly dangerous, from time to time patients do make threats to harm others.

In view of Tarasoff, such a threat directed against a third party can
be very confusing to the therapist in terms of what he must now do. Any
time that a patient harms someone, the immediate question will be raised
as to whether or not the therapist had knowledge that such might occur.
If so, then he might be considered responsible for not having warned the
victim. Since there are many attorneys around, and since such unfortunate mishaps lead to a search for a scapegoat, we can anticipate lawsuits
based on Tarasoff. Whether or not the doctor has such a duty could end
up being a jury question. Since the Tarasoff case was settled out of
court ($35,000), the specific issues never reached a judge or jury. Ini-
tially, many of us believed Tarasoff would not be a real threat, except
in California. However, I am privy to at least one Tarasoff-like case in
Maryland in which a psychiatrist is being sued with the claim that the
doctor had sufficient reason to believe that the plaintiff's life was in danger. In that case the plaintiff was seriously but not fatally injured. A
recent report of a New Jersey trial indicates that the judge agreed with
the majority in the California Tarasoff case and will allow a suit on that
basis (*McIntosh v Milano*, 1979). This opinion will, in all probability, be
appealed. Hopefully, New Jersey's highest court will go along with California's *minority*, which did not believe that the doctor should be held
responsible.

I have received numerous telephone calls from colleagues concerned
about their responsibility because of statements made to them by patients.
In the early 50s Little and Strecker (1956) conducted a survey of members of the Philadelphia Psychiatric Society, with reference to their responsibility to the community in terms of patients who might have committed crimes. At that time the majority of therapists indicated that they
would, in fact, do their best to hospitalize a patient in order to prevent
a crime, but most would not give a warning to a potential victim. They
would also do their very best to have a patient who had committed a
crime turn himself in. Only about half of those surveyed would turn in
a patient who confessed to a very, very serious crime. While I suspect
that the attitude of most psychiatrists prior to Tarasoff would have been
about the same, since Tarasoff, I believe that psychiatrists would be less
reluctant to warn a potential victim.

A recent survey of California psychiatrists indicates that Tarasoff
has had an undesirable effect on psychotherapeutic practice (Stanford
Law Review, 1978). Therapists have become preoccupied with the issue
of dangerousness and find themselves devoting more time to the issue,
both in ferreting out its existence and developing it when present. There
are now more therapists who warn others than there were before Tarasoff.
More therapists discuss the issue of confidentiality than before. It certainly makes good clinical sense to assist the patient in dealing with reality
by indicating to him that you are not going to sit by passively and allow
him to lose control and commit a serious crime. My experience with violent
patients proves that it can be therapeutic to set up a confrontation (without weapons available) between the patient and the intended victim. On
occasion a patient will indicate that he has a gun (a question we rarely
ask!) and is thinking of murdering the spouse or a close relative. Under
such circumstances, it seems to me to be a positive therapeutic element to
indicate to the patient that you are going to warn the potential victim and
see that somebody does something to prevent the patient from harming
himself as well as, and of course, the victim. In view of this, Tarasoff
might not be seen as so onerous. The danger of Tarasoff is that it opens
up another area of invasion of the psychotherapeutic process and burdens

the therapist with concerns that make it more difficult to concentrate on the therapeutic process. One must not only listen with a third ear, but now one needs a fourth to listen for threats that might require a warning.

The confidentiality of the psychotherapeutic relationship has, of course, been invaded by the computer. As more and more data are collected in these infernal machines, the problem may reach crisis proportions. Safeguards to prevent sensitive information from reaching the computer have been developed and yet, for every control that is established, someone has found a means of circumvention. Laws such as the Privacy Act would, on the one hand, seem to attempt to ensure confidentiality. However, other laws such as the Freedom of Information Act would appear to destroy such confidentiality. Certain elements in our federal government, particularly those in law enforcement, have repeatedly attempted to have Congress pass laws that would invade privacy. The efforts of the "Nixon plumbers" to get into Dr. Fielding's office is just one example of the length to which some people will go to obtain information. The recent revelation of the illegal acquisition and sale of information to insurance companies and lawyers by a "medical information bureau" in Denver was certainly blood-chilling. Several bills have been introduced in Congress relative to medical information that, upon review by a noted forensic psychiatrist, Irwin N. Perr (Perr personal communications), appear seriously to invade areas of confidentiality of medical and psychiatric communications.

There is a general acceptance of a social concept of confidentiality in the doctor-patient relationship. However, the law does not allow this *confidential relationship* to easily become a *privileged relationship*. In a privileged relationship, the patient can prevent the doctor from testifying in court. Very few states, in fact, have doctor-patient privilege laws that cover all areas of the doctor-patient relationship, although many states now have privileged communciation laws that protect the relationship between a psychiatrist and the patient. The privilege, of course, is the patient's. He may allow or prevent the therapist from testifying in a legal proceeding as to what was said during this so-called privileged (confidential) relationship.

The development of most privileged communication legislation occurred in the 1960s. These laws were adjusted and fine-tuned during the early and middle 1970s, so that in some states, such as Illinois, "the patient litigant exception" was eliminated. This applies to a situation in which the patient is suing and, therefore, in most states, opens the door or waives his privilege automatically. Illinois has a special provision that does not force the patient automatically to waive his confidential communications if he wishes to be involved in a lawsuit.

In a California case, the Supreme Court of California refused to give Dr. Lifschutz (1972) the right to deciding not to testify when the patient raised the "mental" issue. There was no patient-litigant exception in California. However, the court did call attention to the sensitivity of the psychotherapeutic relationship and indicated that, in interpreting the law, courts should extend as much consideration as possible to the patient and the therapeutic process.

A recent decision by a Virginia trial judge may represent the death knell for conjoint therapy (Washington Post, 1979). The decision stated that the husband had no privilege where the communication was given in the presence of a third party. In this case the third party was the patient's wife, as the communication occurred in conjoint (marriage) therapy.

In legal reasoning this makes perfect sense. A communication given in the presence of a third person cannot be considered *confidential*. But is not conjoint therapy to be considered an exception to such a rule? This case was not appealed for fear that the Court of Appeals would sustain the judge's decision and thereby give this opinion legal precedence. However, since this case has been widely reported in legal newspapers and journals, I am sure it will arise again and eventually reach the appeals level. Perhaps, in order to prevent a crisis before such a ruling gains the stature of precedence, we should work toward corrective legislation lest we see the destruction of conjoint and group therapy. In attempting to treat a couple whose marriage is troubled, can you visualize first warning them that any statements they made in the presence of the other may eventually be used by the spouse in a divorce or custody proceeding, which could occur if the therapeutic efforts to maintain the marriage are not successful? Somehow even the most obtuse must recognize that this would have a dampening effect on any such therapeutic intervention.

We should not feel that this confidentiality crisis is something that concerns psychiatry alone. The Privacy Protection Study Commission in its 1977 report states, "Each time an individual applies for a job, for life or health insurance, for credit, or for financial assistance or services from government, he agrees to relinquish some measure of personal privacy in return for the benefit he seeks. This cannot be helped, but all too often he is asked to sign away far more of his privacy than the situation warrants. . Americans must be concerned about the long-term effect that record-keeping practices can have, not only on relationships between individuals and organizations, but also on the balance of power between government and the rest of society (Daily Record, 1979)." Arthur Miller, a Harvard professor, indicates that data about people is valuable especially if it is derogatory. Investigators of all sorts will pay for such information and, as previously stated, on occasion steal it. One of the real fears is the so-called "buddy system," in which information is traded between friends and agencies and between former government employees and government agencies.

The protection of patients' communications represents a real crisis for psychiatry in the 1980s. I am concerned that there will be further incursions into our attempts to maintain a confidential relationship. Under any form of socialized medicine this could occur to a greater extent than it would if we were to maintain the status quo. Fortunately, vigilance has been maintained by the American Psychiatric Association and other concerned professional groups. Consequently, exceptions, evasions, and loopholes in the confidentiality establishes excellent guidelines and, if implemented, will go a long way toward maintaining confidentiality (Model Law on Confidentiality, 1979).

MALPRACTICE

Is there a malpractice crisis in psychiatry? There is certainly one in medicine. Whether or not there is one in psychiatry remains a question. Attorneys and unhappy plaintiffs are vigorously looking to the mental health field as a possible area of abuse. That professional abuse occurs, there is no question. That patients deserve compensation when they have been negligently wronged also cannot be disputed. The difficult problem, however, is to determine when there has been negligence.

Whenever a patient commits suicide you can be sure that the circumstances surrounding that unfortunate episode will be thoroughly scrutinized by a malpractice attorney. Whether or not the patient's family wished to enter suit, efforts will certainly be made by friends and relatives to encourage them to "do something about it." The general attitude in our society today is that if anything goes wrong, it must have been someone's fault and he should compensate the victim. Fortunately for the mental health profession, it is also recognized that despite our best efforts, we cannot prevent everyone from committing suicide. In some cases, lawsuits involving suicide have been successful and the doctor and/or hospital was judged negligent. Unfortunately, there are no clear-cut standards to be followed in determining what constitutes negligence. A general community standard or even a national standard for the profession may still be rather vague because most situations represent judgment decisions.

If negligence has occurred, it most frequently occurs not at the doctor's hands but as a result of hospital environment and staffing as well as communication of the patient's suicidality. If one is to have suicidal patients on a hospital ward, then it is expected that the ward will have safety screens on the windows, locked doors, and no knives, lighter fluid, or other flammable materials available. On the other hand, the law clearly recognizes that all patients cannot be locked up. There should, however, be some evidence that indicates that the patient is no longer dangerous before he is transferred to a less secure ward. The best judgments are those that are made by two independent individuals and not by one alone.

The fear of malpractice suits can certainly lead to "defensive psychiatry," not too dissimilar from the practice of emergency room medicine where all head injuries receive x-rays whether or not there is a doubt about a skull fracture. This could lead general hospital psychiatrists to the belief that they must try to commit involuntarily all those who attempt suicide whether or not they are currently suicidal. If malpractice suits of this type increase, it could produce a reluctance to transfer patients from closed wards to open wards. (Fortunately I do not think that this type of defensive psychiatry is yet practiced.) Hopefully there will be a reduction in the number of suits that occur because of the public's distaste for such suits and recognition that they raise the cost of medicine. (This may be happening already.) Recent attempts by the medical profession to establish no-fault type insurance has gone a long way toward protecting the public in those rare cases in which the doctor or hospital is negligent.

One area that has not yet been invaded by malpractice suits is psychotherapy. There could be malpractice suits for wrongful, inappropriate, or inadequate psychotherapy. Dawidoff's (1973) book *Psychiatric Malpractice*, published in the early 1970s, has raised that question. Fortunately, such a concept has not caught on with the legal profession. Sexual activity with patients, however, has been an area of legal activity that has resulted in several successful suits.

Product liability (suits against drug companies) has led to an increased look at the utilization of psychotropic medication. Tardive dyskinesia has been recognized as a complication of treatment that may result from negligence. Having well-informed consent from the patient could prevent such suits. Unfortunately, those patients who give their consent forget that they have given it when they have a bad result. (A signed form is not proof that the patient was told and understood everything.) A series of lawsuits successful for the plaintiffs over tardive dyskinesia or other complications of psychotropic medication could represent a very serious crisis for psychiatry because of our reliance upon the psychotropic and antidepressant medications. Because I can remember psychiatry in the late 40s and early 50s without these medications, I cannot conceive of psychiatry in the 80s without the psychotropics or antidepressants.

THE RIGHT TO TREATMENT

Irwin Perr (1979), in a recent guest editorial, says, "In recent years, legislative changes and judicial decisions have drastically altered the management of involuntary patients in governmental institutions. Partly this reflected anxiety about the basic civil rights of those deprived of freedom wherever that might be (e.g. mental hospitals, prisons, juvenile institutions) and partly a concern for how declining public monies were spent with a need for new levels of accountability. It reflected both the growing suspicion of autonomous systems with unchecked power and the numerous philosophical approaches toward the "disadvantaged" of all types." Referring to the right to treatment, he says, "Right to treatment frequently has meant only the opportunity for various groups to assert their claims to the mental health turf and an ill-advised egalitarianism of a poorly rationalized assortment of people who work in mental health settings, all lumped together as 'mental health professionals,' another expression that has spread more darkness than light."

The loss of medical control as a result of some recent decisions has been of prime concern to us. Perr (1979) says, "A common element in recent legal change is the loss of medical input and the legal direction of actual treatment. Some courts are now practicing medicine, doing it badly, and, as the ultimate authority, unchecked without peer review. Many judges recognize the uncomfortable position of trying to be a medical authority based on a scattering of adversarial presentations. As the judge in the Rennie case acknowledged (but did not heed), 'A little knowledge can be dangerous.'"

Perr (1979) has put the issues in clear perspective. The courts in their sincere effort to help our patients have at times made things worse. The increased paper work, committees, advocates, and so on have not really solved the problem, although these efforts have caused some improvements. The question that remains is, Could this have been done more cheaply and efficiently in some other way? I doubt it, since I have been convinced by the argument that change in our society is slow and costly. Next, I would have to wonder, how can one measure some of the changes that supposedly have come about? We see examples describing poor conditions the patients live under in the community as compared to the poor conditions that they lived under in the hospital. Unfortunately, the patients have little to say about this. We also have not had adequate input into many of these decisions. Initially we had very little input because we had inadequate legal representation. Most recently, the sophistication of the representative of the state, the attorneys general, has been greatly improved. In addition, more psychiatrists are beginning to take a more sanguine view of the simple solutions that were promised to us by the mental health bar. At first their idea sounded splendid. Our patients would get better care because they would force the states, through the courts, to furnish more money. We didn't get much money, however. What we got instead were hearings, trials, regulations, individual treatment plans, and so on. Would an equal amount of human effort have produced better results through lobbying of legislatures for more funds by local mental health associations? Would patients' liberty and rights have been protected just as well?

THE RIGHT TO REFUSE TREATMENT

This issue has caused a problem that has, in theory, the potential of creating an overwhelming crisis in psychiatry. In practice, there are indications that it may represent a tempest in a teapot, in that very few

patients really desire to refuse medication since they wish to be well and
the medication helps to accomplish this. This is not to say that some
patients are not overmedicated and should not have their medications reduced. The Rennie (1979) case is a perfect example, however, of the
court stepping into a situation in which it apparently is ill-equipped to
decide despite the testimony that is produced. Judge Bazelon believed
that there should be no problem in having a jurist hear testimony and
to make a decision based on that testimoney. However, we know that it
is exceedingly difficult to make clinical judgments with the type of time
schedule that is inherent in the judicial system. Certainly all psychiatric
out-patients have the right to refuse treatment. Some very disturbed
patients, in fact chronically psychotic schizophrenic patients, do this,
causing a great deal of difficulty for themselves and society. Generally
speaking, these patients eventually learn that they have to keep taking
their medicine, despite the fact that it may have undesirable side effects,
or else they are going to end up in the hospital or in jail. Unfortunately,
in the process, great suffering may occur to them and their families or,
even worse, to some stranger who is assaulted or seriously injured by
some unmedicated psychotic. This is a crisis in view of the fact that it
is so difficult to make clear to the law that mentally ill individuals have
an incapacity to form rational judgments.

The most recent Rennie (1979) case ruling establishes a system for
informing patients of all side reactions, complications, and so on. It also
utilizes advocates to help patients understand their right to refuse treatment. It will be curious to see how the efforts to obtain informed consent
and the efforts of advocates to inform patients of their right to refuse
will balance out. Will there be so many refusing patients that the hospital
will be bedlam? Will only 5 to 10 percent of the patients refuse, but take
up so much professional time that there will be no time left for the complaint patients? One hope that I have is that the consent committee's
hearing officers, if furnished sufficient followup, will develop clinical
judgment. I suspect that within the next several years we will see the
further development of the staff conference for review and decision making.
A new approach might be that individuals from other disciplines, such as
the clergy, attorneys, and lay persons, may be present to assist us in
looking at the situation from a different angle. This may help prevent
some of the self-fulfilling prophecies that influence our decisions and
planning. I feel that, as some of the impractical approaches of the human
rights movement are corrected, a process will be developed by which those
patients who are unhappy with their treatment regimen or who have not
shown an adequate response will have a complete review of their treatment
with the development of alternate plans. What this means of course is
more staff for hospitals and clinics, with more time to look at such situations in detail. Hopefully, this will be the final result when it is no
longer necessary to spend time and money defending lawsuits.

COMMITMENT

We have hung ourselves on our own petard in terms of the concept of
dangerousness as a criterion for commitment. We knew who was dangerous
when we applied *our* standards. However, we did not utilize a criminal-
legal definition of dangerousness, which has subsequently been used by
the courts. Liberty is one of the fundamental pillars of our democratic
society and no one would want to change that. However, there is also no
question that there are mentally ill people who are incapable of managing
themselves in the community without untold suffering to themselves and
others, who nevertheless do not meet the criminal criteria of dangerous-

ness. The law is beginning to recognize this. The Supreme Court (*Addington v Texas*, 1979), in establishing a standard of proof for voluntary commitment, chose the middle ground of the three possible tests — "clear and convincing evidence" — indicating the court's recognition that dealing with commitment of the mentally ill is not the same as dealing with the finding of guilt of criminals. The Supreme Court further upheld the parents' right to commit in the case of *Parham v J.L. and J.R.* (1979), recognizing that full legal-type commitment hearings for children were counterproductive. We need to get away from the dangerous concept promulgated by the Supreme Court in *Donaldson*, when it held that a mentally ill individual could not be committed against his will merely because he was ill, but that the would have to be either dangerous or unable to care for himself in the community.

There are several different factors that must be considered when we apply such standards. Alan Stone (1975) believes that there should be a clear diagnosis of mental illness; that the person should be involved in what might be considered a major distress, that is, an incapacity to function outside of the hospital in any reasonable fashion; that treatment is in fact available; and that the diagnosed illness impaired the person's ability to make a treatment judgment, that is, he is refusing treatment as a result of his illness and a reasonable man would accept such treatment (hospitalization). I suspect that Stone's criteria might even be watered down as time goes on, since I wonder whether the 1980s might not show a regression or return to a more paternalistic attitude toward commitment. Loren Roth, M.D. (1979) has recently described two commitment schemes. One, under parens patriae circumstances, would not require really dangerous behavior but be time-limited, and patients could not refuse reasonable short-term treatment (not competent for treatment to be determined at time of commitment). Longer commitments (police power) would require truly dangerous (to self or others) behavior and would be for longer periods.

Space limitations have allowed me to describe only a few of the many areas of the practice of psychiatry that have been affected by recent actions of the law. There are many other areas that may seem more important to those closely involved. We can be certain that there will be further changes, shifts, and alterations. There is more to come in the areas of the right to refuse treatment, consent, confidentiality, and Tarasoff. There will be substantial revisions of some of the legal positions once we have the opportunity to clarify the problems and present our opinions, ideas, and data in a clear and consistent fashion. The Judicial Action Commission of the American Psychiatric Association has become involved in the more important cases and has produced briefs that have presented the patients' therapeutic needs and the psychiatrists' problems in a manner that has allowed the courts to arrive at more reasonable decisions.

I firmly believe that all of us want the best for our patients. All of us want to prevent suffering and to help patients become autonomous and free human beings. It is now more clear than ever that this cannot be accomplished alone by either psychiatry or the law. While each profession wishes to improve mankind's conditions, we operate on parallel roads that seem never to meet, and certainly will not if either prevails to a greater degree than the other. My hope and belief is that we can eventually produce an amalgam that will allow psychiatrists to practice unfettered, and allow our patients the maximum freedom and liberty, along with the best opportunity and conditions to recover from their illness.

REFERENCES

Addington v Texas. 47, U.S.L.W. 4473, 1979.
183 Daily Record No. 36. August 18, 1979.
Dawidoff, D.J. *The Malpractice of Psychiatrists.* Springfield,
    Charles C. Thomas, 1973.
Klein, J. Supreme Court Decision Poses Broad Threat to Confidentiality.
    Legal Aspects of Medical Practice 7:42-44, 1979.
Lifschutz, J.E. 467, P.2d 557, 1972.
Little, R.B. and Strecker, E.A. Moot Questions in Psychiatric Ethics,
    Amer. J. Psychiat. 113:5:455-460, 1956.
McIntosh v Milano. NJ Super Ct., Law Div., Bergen City, June 12, 1979.
    The Criminal Law Reporter 25:16, 1979.
Model Law on Confidentiality of Health and Social Service Records. *Amer.*
    J. Psychiat. 136:1, 1979.
Parham v J.L. 47, U.S.L.W. 4740, 1979.
Perr, I.N. Personal communication. Re: H.R. 2979 and H.R. 3444.
Perr, I.N. Sologans (guest editorial). *Psychiatric News* 16:15, 1979.
Rappeport, J.R. Rights. Speech 8th Annual Institute Hospital and
    Community Psychiatry, Atlanta, Ga., Sept. 20, 1976. Reported
    in *Hospital & Community Psychiatry* 28, p. 36; and Balance of
    Patients' Rights-Care Argued. *Psychiatric News,* 11:20, 1976.
Rennie v Klein. Preliminary Injuection. Original Filed Sept. 14, 1979
    in the U.S. District Court for the District of N.J.
Roth, L.H. A commitment law for patients, doctors, and lawyers. *Amer.*
    J. Psychiat. 136:91121-1127, 1979.
Stanford Law Review 31:121, 1978, pp. 165-190. Where the public peril
    begins: A survey of psychotherapists to determine the effects of
    Tarasoff.
Stone, A.A. Mental Health and Law: A System in Transition, Crime and
    Delinquency Issues; A Monograph Series. NIMH, DHEW Publication
    No. (ADM) 75-176, 1975.
Tarasoff v Regents of the University of California. 551, P.2d 334, 1976.
Washington Post. March 19, 1979. (Circuit Court Judge Richard J.
    Jamborsky, Arlington, Va.), Lawyers Upset at Ruling Psychiatrist
    Must Testify.
Zurcher v Stanford Daily. U.S. Law Week, 46 LW 4546, 1978.

NOTE:

AN ADDENDUM TO THIS CHAPTER WAS
SUBMITTED AS THE BOOK WAS GOING
TO PRESS AND APPEARS ON PAGES 143-144.

6

Informed Consent: Elements for Crisis

Richard C.W. Hall
Earl R. Gardner

The elements involved in defining informed consent represent a prototypic model that highlights the many forces impinging upon the field of psychiatry:

- The goal of protecting patients is worthy and cannot be easily assailed.
- A mechanism for patient protection must be established.
- It is assumed that the competent physician will participate in the protection of his patients.
- A regulator is needed for "those few physicians who would violate" the guidelines.
- Finally, a hearing board (be it committee or court) is necessary to arbitrate disputes.

Within this framework, and based upon the assumption that the patient may be injured by physician negligence, or that the patient must be protected from the non-patient-related goals of the physician (be they monetary gain or research aggrandizement), a series of ombudsmen as impressive as the long grey line have emerged. Governmental secretaries, bureaucrats at all levels, lawyers, judges, citizens' rights groups- and left-wing social advocacy groups, nurses, social workers, feminists, right to life groups, and members of the media have all volunteered their special insights and skills to protect patients from their physicians. All are willing to insert themselves between doctor and patient in the doctor-patient relationship. In so doing, some have questioned whether they create more harm for more people than they could ever hope to cure (Cole, 1977; Meyer, 1977; Robins, 1977, Gray, 1977).

Before addressing the dilemmas created for the field by the conflicting doctrine of informed consent, let us, at least briefly, try to sketch the evolution of our current dilemma.

INFORMED CONSENT FROM THERE TO HERE

One of the earliest malpractice cases on record related to informed consent. In 1767, Slater sued Baker and Stapleton (1978) after Baker had put "a heavy steel thing that had teeth on the plantiff's leg which broke that leg. And for three or four months afterwards the plantiff was still very ill and bad of it." The case resolved to the fact that Baker wanted to experiment with this new instrument and was found guilty of having experimented without detailing in advance the risks and benefits

Note: Modified and updated from a paper published in the American Journal of Forensic Psychiatry (Hall, 1978); parts reproduced with permission.

of the procedure. The court ruled that he could not merely proceed as
he thought best. With few legal exceptions, however, during the next
150 years, doctors did proceed as they thought best. Because of their
position in the community, few challenged their motives. However, in
1945, four physicians were hanged by the neck until dead at Nuerenberg.
They had been responsible for perpetrating "inhuman and grievous crimes
against humanity." The Nuerenberg Code was thus formulated and became a standard, governing the conduct of ethical medical researchers.
Because of the importance of this document, it is reproduced here in its
entirety.

The Nuerenberg Code

1. The voluntary consent of the human subject is absolutely
essential. This means that the person involved should have
legal capacity to give consent, should be so situated as to
be able to exercise free power of choice, without the intervention of any element of force, fraud, deceit, duress,
overreaching, or other ulterior forms of constraint or coercion and should have sufficient knowledge and comprehension of the elements of the subject matter involved as
to enable him to make an understanding and enlightening
decision. This latter element requries that before the
acceptance of an affirmative decision by the experimental
subject, there should be made known to him the nature,
duration, and purpose of the experiment; the method and
means by which it is to be conducted; all inconveniences
and hazards reasonably to be expected; and the effects
upon his health or person which may possibly come from
his participation in the experiment.
     The duty and responsibility of ascertaining the quality
of the consent rests upon each individual who initiates,
directs, or engages in the experiment. It is a personal
duty and responsibility which may not be delegated to
another with impunity.
2. The experiment should be such as to yield fruitful
results for the good of society, unprocurable by other
methods or means of study, and not random and unnecessary in nature.
3. The experiment should be so designed and based on
the results of animal experimentation and a knowledge
of the natural history of the disease or other problems
under study that the anticipated results will justify the
performance of the experiment.
4. The experiment should be so conducted as to avoid
all unnecessary physical and mental suffering and
injury.
5. No experiment should be conducted where there is an
a priori reason to believe that death or disabling injury
will occur: except, perhaps, in those experiments where
the experimental physician also serves as subject.
6. The degree of risk to be taken should never exceed
that determined by the humanitarian importance of the
problem to be solved by the experiment.
7. Proper preparations should be made and adequate
facilities provided to protect the experimental subject
against even remote possibilities of injury, disability,
or death.

8. The experiment should be conducted only by scientifically qualified persons. The highest degree of skill and care should be required through all stages of the experiment, of those who conduct or engage in the experiment.

9. During the course of the experiment, the human subject should be at liberty to bring the experiment to an end if he has reached the physical or mental state where continuation of the experiment seems to him to be impossible.

10. During the course of the experiment, the scientist in charge must be prepared to terminate the experiment at any state, if he has probable cause to believe, in the exercise of the good faith, superior skill, and careful judgement required of him, that a continuation of the experiment is likely to result in the injury, disability, or death to the experimental subject.

The Nuerenberg Code clearly defined that all risks must be detailed to a subject, regardless of any psychological risks such disclosure would create for that particular patient. Many physicians were concerned by this element of the Code, since they felt that itemizing all risks to a patient might potentially place him in psychological jeopardy. Because of this concern, the 1954 Declaration of Helsinki provided the following: "If at all possible, consistent with a patient's psychology, the doctor should obtain the patient's freely given consent after the patient has been given a full explanation." The physician now found himself bound by charges of paternalism if he withheld information, or of callousness if he provided information that subsequently emotionally damaged his patient. In 1962, the United States Food, Drug and Cosmetic Act was amended to include a provision that any investigator must obtain the *informed consent* of the individual to whom a new drug was to be administered. In 1966, Beecher's report, Ethics in Clinical Research, shocked the medical community and was widely publicized in the lay press. He gave 22 examples of unethical or questionably ethical medical research conducted by established researchers from major academic institutions and hospitals within the United States. Many of the subjects of this research had never had the experimental risks explained to them. Furthermore, literally hundreds of them had never been told that they were participating in experiments from which substantial personal harm might occur. These reports were not at all dissimilar to recent newspaper stories concerning schizophrenic patients having experimental adrenalectomies performed on them without their full knowledge of the risks involved. In 1967, following Beecher's report, the Federal Food and Drug Administration revised its consent policy and instructed investigators and sponsors of research that they must obtain *"knowledgeable informed consent"* as a prerequisite to any human investigational work. Two years later, in 1969, the National Institute of Health for the first time required any institution that received federal grants to establish committees to ensure that *proper informed consent* be obtained prior to beginning any human experimentation.

Informed consent was defined by HEW as follows: "Informed consent means the knowing consent of an individual or his legally authorized representative, so situated as to be able to exercise free power of choice without undue inducement of any element of force, fraud, deceit, duress or other forms of constraint or coercion. The basic elements of information necessary for such consent included: (1) a fair explanation of the procedures to be followed and their purposes, including identification of any procedures that are experimental; (2) a description of any attendant discomforts and risks reasonably to be expected; (3) a description of any benefits reasonably to be expected; (4) a disclosure of any appropriate alternative procedures that might be advantageous for the subjects; (5) an offer to answer any inquiries concerning the procedure, and (6) an instrument that the person is free to withdraw his consent and to discontinue participation in the project or activity at any time without prejudice to the subject (Weinberger, 1974)." Section 46.2 of HEW Policy, subparagraph B3, adds the following: *"Legally effective* informed consent will be obtained by *adequate* and *appropriate* methods in accordance with the provisions of this part."

As one can readily see, these "governmental provisions" have protected those making the laws from undue attack, but have left the field investigator with the burden of defining what is "legally effective." If an investigator knew what legal test would be applied to define whether a consent was legally effective, he could then gauge his compliance. Unfortunately, no one can know which legal test will be applied, as many doctrines can be evoked, including the "general knowledge doctrine," the "locality role," the "materiality test," the "full and complete disclosure role," or the "subjective and objective test of disclosure" (Hall, 1978).

Even if an investigator knew which test would be applied, he would still have to contend with the issue of whether a particular psychiatric patient *could* give informed consent. The legal guidelines defining this question were originally put forth in 1914 by Justice Cardozo: "Every human being of adult years and sound mind has a right to determine what shall be done with his own body" (*Schloendorff v Society of N.Y. Hospital*, 1914). By implication, the Justice suggests that individuals who are not of sound mind do not have the right to determine what can be done with their own body, even if they are fully informed. The current federal regulations seem to concur on this point (Weinberger, 1974): "The department (HEW) now proposes that in addition to the protection afforded generally to all subjects of research, development, and related activity, supported by the department by virtue of part 46, further protective measures should be provided for those subjects of research whose capability of providing informed consent is, or may be, absent or limited." Sub-part E of these regulations requires additional protection for the rights of the mentally ill, the mentally retarded, the emotionally disturbed, and the senile, who are confined to institutions, whether by voluntary or involuntary commitment. "Such persons, by the very nature of their disabilities, may be severely limited in their capacity to provide informed consent for their participation in research."

Since individuals suffering from mental infirmity or illness may not be able to give informed consent, federal regulations go on to further define a system for ensuring their protection (Weinberger, 1974). "The term, 'legal guardian,' is used to replace the term, 'legally authorized representative.'" This change clearly states that the federal position is that only a court-appointed legal guardian is empowered to give informed consent for research purposes in the case of a mentally incompetent individual. Thus, we can see that the protection of the individual has, in fact, come full circle to the point that, legally speaking, psychiatric research today is possible only in the strictest sense of the word, when conducted with psychiatric patients who have been rendered legally incompetent by a court of law and have had a guardian appointed who can then legally authorize their participation in a research study.

What about the issue of informed consent and routine treatment? Research, it can be argued, is a relatively circumscribed area that requires heightened guidelines for subject protection. The informed consent doctrine, on the other hand, also applies to a patient's knowledge of proposed treatment. Here we must look to case law. Perhaps the most important recent decision is the case of *Canterbury v Spence* (1972; Knapp, 1975), which was decided in 1972 in the District of Columbia Circuit Court of Appeals. The case was cited as being "a revolution in malpractice law," which represented "a departure without precedent to a standard requiring that 'everything' be told to the patient" (Rosenberg, 1973; Rubsamen, 1973; Breckler, 1973). The court affirmed, in upholding the standards of *Wall v Brim* (1943), that "due care normally demands that the physician warn a patient of any risk to his well-being that the contemplated therapy may involve." It stated that the particular form of treatment undertaken is the prerogative of the patient, not of the physician, and that, consequently, all therapeutic alternatives and hazards must be delineated to the patient for him to make such choice. Justice Robertson in this case struck down the majority rule, stating that the standard of disclosure based on the custom of physicians practicing in the community did not provide adequate protection for the patient's rights, since the patient should not be dependent for information upon "relevent professional tradition."

The Canterbury court ruled that, once an issue of medical treatment had been raised, the physician had a duty to disclose. The extent of that duty was defined as providing the information necessary for the patient to make an "intelligent decision." The court further ruled that the standard for that decision must be "measured by the patient's need and that need is the information material to the decision." The court believed that the physician would be liable if there was "unreasonably inadequate communication," using as a standard

physician might have communicated to his patients. The court said that all side effects and complications must be pointed out if they had either a high probability of occurrence or a slight probability of occurrence, but were associated with significant harm. Thus, the significance of risk was determined by knowledge of a procedure's ability to cause harm, that is, either the "incidence of injury" or "the degree of harm" that could reasonably be expected.

Although Canterbury was applauded as a standard, at least seven major cases that occurred subsequent to it have been decided in a somewhat different manner. Four have followed, with minor variation, the Canterbury rule, while three have totally rejected it. In *Wilkinson v Versey* (1972), the Rhode Island Supreme Court proposed a doctrine of individuality and stated that the doctor-patient relationship was a one-to-one affair. This court upheld the principle that what was reasonable disclosure in one instance might not be reasonable in another, and that this variability negated the need of the plantiff to show what other doctors might tell their patients.

The California Supreme Court, in *Cobbs v Grant* (1972), cautioned the physician that he must fulfill a two-fold duty to disclose. First, he must explain any risk of death or serious harm, *no matter how remote*, as well as outlining in lay terms any complications that could occur. Second, he must inform his patient of any additional information "as a skilled practitioner would provide under similar circumstances." Thus, the Supreme Court of California imposed a community standard rule, in addition to the rule of Canterbury, for its jurisdiction. In deciding what was material, the California court said that information is material to a patient's decision if not only he, but also any reasonable and prudent person, would have refused treatment had such risk and consequences been made known. Other cases bearing on this topic, (*Fogal v Genesee Hospital* (1973), *Frogun v Fruchturan* (1973), *Funke v Fieldman* (1973), *Nathanson v Kline* (1960), *Zebarth v Swedish Hospital Medical*

Center (1972), and *Collins v Stoh* (1972)) all suggest that the physician's duty to disclose is predicted on the patient's right to give informed consent for a given procedure. Yet, many of these decisions predicate their standards on contradictory case law. What does seem to hold is that all procedures that have a small possibility of occurrence and are related to a slight magnitude of harm need not be enumerated, while procedures that, no matter how small their probability of occurrence, are related to a major magnitude of harm must be disclosed. In addition, the individual must have a "substantive capacity" to understand any potential risks and must be able to provide written and *"legally effective"* informed consent. The courts have generally agreed that infants, children, legal minors, and mental incompetents may be, in general, impaired and thus incapable of giving "informed consent."

In situations where psychiatrists do insist on guardianship, recent court decisions suggest that even a properly appointed guardian may not be able to consent to certain procedures (Richardson, 1973). There are also cases which hold that guardians cannot consent to their ward's involvement in research projects that are not specifically designed to benefit them (Chayet, 1978).

The incorporation of informed consent statutes into criminal law has already occurred in the states of Massachussets and Louisiana. In Massachussets it is a criminal offense for a physician to fail to get informed consent for any research project involving the use of a controlled or dangerous substance, which in that state includes by definition any prescription drug (Chayet, 1978). Louisiana makes it an offense, carrying a penalty of up to 20 years at hard labor, for a physician to fail to get informed consent in treatment-research situations (Chayet, 1978).

The physician may also be sued for fully informing his patient if such information produces injury. Chayet (1978) reports the case of a physician who was concerned about informing his patients, lest he be sued for not providing informed consent. He consequently detailed all of the possible hazards of a coronary bypass operation to an individual with coronary insufficiency. After the patient left the doctor's office he died. His family brought suit against the surgeon for causing the death by wrongfully securing the patient's informed consent.

This "damned if you do, damned if you don't" situation suggests that some social process is operative and productive of conflict, since the courts routinely, if belatedly, reflect society's concerns with their rulings.

AN ANALYSIS OF ROLE AND MODEL

Traditionally, the doctor-patient relationship assumes that the physician is predominantly interested in the welfare and improvement of the ill patient; that he has expertise and knowledge to apply in the direction of cure; that he is honor-bound to respect the dignity and prerogatives of the patient; and that his patient wishes, by virture of his sick role, to be cured or to have his pain and suffering ameliorated. The physician in this paradigm assumes responsibility for the direction of the patient's life, and in so doing relieves him of certain societal expectations and obligations. The patient is entitled to assume the sick role under the care of a physician until such time as the physician certifies that he is able to return to his normal place in society. The physician's ability to alter the patient's social role and function is a normally expected concomitant of the doctor-patient relationship. If, however, it is assumed that the physician no longer represents the best interest of the patient, or if his motives for altering the patient's societal role become suspect, then all powers and prerogatives that he exercises can be seen as abusive rather

than helpful. Consequently, once the intent of the physician's intervention is challenged, a need arises to protect the patient from the power of
the physician. In the case of the psychiatrist, the physician's potential
destructive power (vis a vis commitment, loss of civil liberties, psychosurgery, the administration of drugs, etc.) takes on frightening proportions in the public's mind.

Since the physician's role is accorded by society, based on society's
expectations of cure, the doctor-patient relationship can also be jeopar-
dized or made suspect if the physician is felt to offer hoax rather than
remedy. The charlatan is not entitled to the prerogatives of the healer.
The psychiatrist has, unfortunately, been put in the position of charlatan
by offering more than he can deliver and by acting as an agent of the
state. In this latter role, he has been seen by many as the oppressor of
the mentally ill rather than as their guardian. Such a position nullifies
societal support of his role and makes him a legitimate target for patient
advocate groups.

Many of the problems defined above do not relate exclusively to the
field of psychiatry. Strong social pressure is being applied in a systematic fashion to bring to public awareness or, as some feel, to make the
public erroneously believe that a physician's behavior is not entirely
determined by altruism and professionalism. Reports of excessive numbers of unnecessary operations, petty squabbling and political warfare
between physicians and hospitals, professional self-aggrandizement,
massive earnings by physicians, Medicare fraud, and the declining availability of even moderate quality health care have all tarnished the physician's image of respectability. The ultimate end of these facts or frictions,
depending upon one's point of view, is increased government regulation
and control of the health care system (or industry) in the United States.
For good or ill, informed consent standards and laws will play a key role
in defining the nature of this governmental control of medicine in America.

FUTURE IMPLICATIONS AND EFFECTS
OF INFORMED CONSENT DOCTRINE

The case law changes defining informed consent will have an impact
both on the practice of psychiatry and on the clinician's ability to conduct human research. In the research arena, permissible research will
be defined by an analysis of risk-benefit ratio, the nature of the participating subjects, and the quality and nature of the informed consent obtained. Many institutions have already moved toward committees to certify
the risk-benefit ratio as acceptable and to screen participating research
subjects. The use of surrogate consentors, as advocated by Frost (1975)
and others, is becoming increasingly popular. In fact, the next decade
may bring to us a whole new class of professionals who are univerally
educated to function as consentors, and who, if bureaucratic practice fol-
lown, will develop their own specialty board and professional society.
These individuals may be institutionally defined to function as translators
between patients and physicians. They would increase the protection
afforded human subjects participating in research, but would also do great
harm by interposing yet another agent between the doctor and his patient.

The surrogate consent system was in part initially applauded because
it controlled for physician's abuse of information and protected patients
from being forced to provide "informed consent" in clinicial settings where
they were anxious or dependent. Such a model, however, assumes that
the doctor-patient relationship itself destroys the patient's ability to consent. The implications of such an assumption are far-reaching, since it

suggests that no matter how well-meaning the physician, he can never deal with a truly free subject.

The new disclosure doctrines will make physicians more conscious of their legal requirments and thus increase their practice of defensive medicine. Medical costs will continue to rise and physician availability diminish, which will in turn prompt tougher health care legislation (Bernstein, 1975). Although legislative efforts will certainly continue and increase, their success for facilitating useful research while protecting human subjects will, in legislative approach has already plateaued. One cannot legislate ethics any more than one can legislate common sense and good judgment. Other trends that may develop are concerted efforts by journals to bar the publication of unethical studies and thereby diminish the professional incentive for less than well-founded research. Perhaps we will also see a change in the curriculums of our medical schools, as the federal government once again begins to question the capitation funds that it supplies to these institutions. In ensuing decades we may also see an increased emphasis on courses in clinical research, legal medicine, and medical ethics.

The long-term effect of current trends of informed consent litigation may be to provide significant barriers to research in psychopharmacology, as has been suggested by Jonathan Cole (1977). Cole elegantly argues that the changes in public policy and law over the last several years have made the development of new psychopharmacological agents progressively more difficult, with each new layer of regulation impeding the progress of legitimate investigators and increasing the cost of drug development. The attacks by scientologists on the Missouri Institute of Psychiatry and the legal aid group on research at the Lafayette Clinic have resulted in both of these institutions abandoning, at least for a time, drug research.

The politicalization of review functions is also likely to occur, as present regulations require institutional review boards to be staffed by totally disinterested and unpaid citizen members. Very often the findings of such review structures are determined by board politics and philosophies, rather than scientific fact. Concerns already exist that such bodies have impaired the scientists' legitimate right and freedom to inquire. As Meyer (1977) points out, research investigators in the biomedical and behavioral sciences have been placed in the position of defending their work in an adversary climate. He argues strongly that "subject's rights" not be viewed only in a legalistic context, but also in the context of not harming the patient. The ability to conduct followup studies has also been severely affected by these regulations, particularly in the area of child research (Robins, 1977). The sociologist Gray (1977) raises concern directed at the three emerging functions of human subject review committees: (1) the protection of institutions; (2) the judgment of research in terms of its social policy impact; and (3) the approval of research from the standpoint of "community acceptability." He raises questions as to the destructive effects that politicalization may have on the overall treatment of the psychiatric patient.

In closing, one is left to consider Laforet's (1976) ultimate analysis of the problem. "In the final analysis, regardless of whether society or the medical profession or the law wants it that way, the best and probably only guarantee of a patient's or subject's rights is the integrity of his physician."

REFERENCES

Beecher, H.K. Ethics in clinical research. *N. Engl. J. Med.* 274:1354-1360, 1966.

Bernstein, J.E. Ethical considerations in human experimentation. *J. Clin Pharmac.* 15:579-570, 1975.

Breckler, I.A., Price, E.M., and Shore, S. Informed consent: A new majority position. *J. Leg. Med.* 1(3):37, 1973.

Canterbury v Spence. 464 F.2d 772, D.C. Cir., 1972; See also Informed Consent Landmark, 1(2) *J. Legal Med.* 16, 1973.

Chayet, N.L. Can Informed Consent be obtained from a Psychiatric Patient? Patient Surrogates: A Possibility of Improving the Present System. In Brady and Brodie, H.K.H. (eds.) Controversy in Psychiatry. W.B. Saunders, Philadelphia, 1978, pp. 997-1007.

Cobbs v Grant. 8 Cal. 3d 299, 104 Cal. Rptr. 505, 502 p. 2d 1, 1972.

Cole, J.O. Research barriers in psychopharmacology. *Am. J. Psychiat.* 134:8:896-898, 1977.

Collins v Stoh. 503 p.2d 36, 1972.

Fogal v Genesee Hospital. 41 A.D. 168 344 N.Y.S. 2d 552, 1973.

Frogun v Truchgturan. 58 Wis. 2d 596, 207 N.W. 2d 297, 1973.

Frost, N.C. A surrogate system for informed consent. *JAMA* 233:7:800-803, 1975.

Funke v Fieldman, 212 Kan. 524, 512, p. 2d 539, 1973.

Gray, B.H. The functions of human subjects review committees. *Am. J. Psychiat.* 134:8:907-910, 1977.

Hall, R.C.W. Psychiatric research — the psychotic patient and informed consent: Through the looking glass. *Am. J. Forensic Psychiat.* 1:1:42-63, 1978.

Knapp, T.A. and Huff, R.L. Emerging trends in the physician's duty to disclose: An update of *Canterbury v Spence. J. of Leg. Med.* V.3:1, p. 41-45, 1975.

Laforet, E.G. The fiction of informed consent. *JAMA* 235:15:1579-1585, 1966.

Meyer, R.E. Subjects' rights, freedom of inquiry, and the future of research in the addictions. *Am. J. Psychiat.* 134:8:899-903, 1977.

Nathanson v Kline. 186 Kan. 393, 350 p 2d 1093, 1960.

Richardson. 248 S.O. 2V 185, La. App., 1973.

Robins, L.N. Problems in follow-up studies. *Am. J. Psychiat.* 134:8:904-907, 1977.

Rosenberg, A.R. Informed consent — the latest threat? *J. Leg. Med.* V.17, 1973.

Rubsamen, D.S. Informed consent: New decisions create new impacts. 1(2) *J. Leg. Med.* 6, 1973.

Schloendorff v Society of N.Y. Hospital. 211 N.Y., 125, 129, 105, N.E. 92, 1914.

Slater v Baker and Stapleton. C.B. 95 Eng. Rep. 860, 1767. Cited in Chayot, N.L. Patient surrogates. Possibility of improvement. Controversary in Psychiatry, J.P. Brady, H.K. Bordie, (eds.). Philadelphis: W.B. Saunders Co., 1978, p. 998.

Wall v Brim. 138 F.2d 478 5th Cir., 1943.

Weinberger, C.W. *Fed Reg.,* V.39:165, Friday, August 23, p. 306-348, 1974a.

Weinberger, C.W. *Fed Reg.,* V.39:165, Friday, August 23, p. 306-349, 1974b.

Weinberger, C.W. *Fed. Reg.* V.39:105, Thursday, May 30, p. 18917, Sec. 46.2 (B) (3) and Sec. 46.3 (C), 1974.

Wilkinson v Versey. 295 A 2d 676, 1972.

Zebarth v Swedish Hospital Medical Center. 81 Wash. 2d 12, 499 p 2d 1, 1972.

7

Psychotherapy: Alive or Dead?

Jerome D. Frank

The short answer to the question posed by the title of this chapter that comes to mind is: Both. Depending on one's point of view, one can select evidence to show that psychotherapy is either in vigorous health or, if not dead, is moribund. This is because psychotherapy has never simultaneously been in greater demand and under more vigorous attack. In the last two decades, psychotherapy has been undergoing a continuous explosion, and the end does not seem to be in sight. Its targets have spread from individuals to families and groups, and now whole neighborhoods. Methods range from traditional interviews to tickling, nude marathons, and elaborate rituals of meditation; practitioners have broken the bounds of the traditional disciplines and now include many whose only training is having undergone the therapy they offer to others, or who are simply fellow sufferers. The settings in which therapy is conducted have burst out of hospitals and offices, into living rooms, motels, and resorts — and new psychotherapies spring up almost overnight like mushrooms. Wolberg, in his latest edition of *The Technique of Psychotherapy*, takes about 200 pages simply to briefly describe the therapies now extant (Wolberg, 1977).

This lush overgrowth, of course, is in response to public demand, which seems insatiable. Individuals are not only flocking to psychotherapies in droves, but are frantically searching for solutions to their personal problems in self-help books, which repeatedly make best-seller lists. At the same time, influential psychiatrists and laymen are claiming that, at best, psychotherapy is a delusion shared by patients and therapists and, at worst, an expensive fraud purporting to treat normal human unhappiness by calling it mental illness (Gross, 1978).

To resolve this apparent paradox, this chapter will first seek to define and describe psychotherapy, and then will examine the evidence with respect to its effectiveness, with the aim of reaching a satisfactory answer to the question posed by the title.

The term "psychotherapy" refers to treatment of psychologically caused distress and diability by psychological means — that is, through symbolic communication. So defined, it would cover all the activities mentioned above, as well as others. These can all be encompassed by a definition that considers psychotherapy to be an emotionally charged interaction in which a trained, socially sanctioned healer, often with the participation of a group of other sufferers, seeks to relieve a sufferer's distress and disability through a systematic set of activities, guided by a more or less clearly articulated conceptual scheme. The main therapeutic tool is symbolic communication, usually by words but sometimes including bodily activities that carry a large symbolic overload.

Psychotherapy defined this broadly would have to include, at one extreme, activities such as biofeedback and, at the other, transcendental religious cults. Biofeedback is a form of psychotherapy in that it is essentially instrument-aided Yoga. That is, Yogi can accomplish by strictly psychological means everything that biofeedback does with the use of a machine. At the other extreme, while the conceptual framework of religious cults is based on transcendental sanctions, they do have powerful psychological healing effects on many adherents, and these always involve symbolic interactions with the cult leader.

Other therapies involve groups consisting of patients, ex-patients, or potential patients with similar difficulties who have banded together to help themselves, such as AA, consciousness raising groups, and those covered by the term "human potential movement." While none of these is defined as psychotherapy by its participants, and many in the first two categories lack a trained leader, their philosophies and procedures frequently resemble those of more traditional group therapies. The fact that most of their participants have been or are simultaneously receiving formal psychotherapy confirms that many of the same principles are involved (Lieberman, 1977).

Confining ourselves for simplicity's sake to those procedures that are in the mainstream of group or individual psychotherapy, these are based on two underlying philosophies: the scientific and the existential. The basic assumption underlying all forms of "scientific" psychotherapy is that man is part of the animal kingdom, which, like all of nature, is ruled by natural laws. Therefore, human behavior, thinking, and feeling are determined and constrained by genetic endowment, biologically based needs, and the effects of beneficial and harmful environmental influences. Insofar as they are correctable by psychotherapy, distress and disability are caused by warping early-life experiences, either the presence of noxious ones or the absence of ones that are essential for normal development. These influences result in maladaptive attitudes and behavior, which are then self-perpetuating. Therapeutic procedures grounded on scientific principles seek to combat these maladaptive patterns and encourage more appropriate ones.

Scientific therapies can be roughly grouped in accordance with whether they place their main emphasis on the cognitive, affective, or behavioral aspects of human functioning. Since all three are always involved, this division is a matter of emphasis only. Therapies emphasizing cognition and emotion are largely developments of aspects of Freudian theory, which was based on clinical experience. Freudian psychoanalysis emphasized cognitions by stressing the curative effect of insight brought about by interpretations of the historical causes of one's difficulties. The healing emotional component of psychoanalysis was thought to be catharsis, the reliving with full emotional intensity of the traumatic early experiences supposedly responsible for the patient's current difficulties. Springing from Freudian theory, some therapies, such as primal scream therapy (Janov, 1970), have heavily emphasized the curative effect of abreaction. Others have stressed efforts to modify a patient's cognitions about himself and others (Beck, 1976; Ellis, 1962).

The behavioral emphasis in psychotherapy springs from the contributions of another genius, Ivan Pavlov, and later from E. L. Thorndike and B. F. Skinner. Behavior therapists claim to have a scientific basis for their procedures because they are allegedly based on animal experiments. The extent to which these procedures have actually been derived from experiments rather than clinical experience remains debatable. Although some behavior therapists would claim that behavior therapy is distinct from psychotherapy, the therapeutic components of behavior therapies overlap widely with those of the other forms of scientific psychotherapy. Behavioral therapies seek to shape behavior through modifying its instigators and consequences. Those deriving mainly from Pavlov have stressed the extinction of pathological emotional reactions such as phobias through eliciting them simultaneously with reactions that are incompatible with them — for example, relaxation (Wolpe and Lazarus, 1966). Those that derive from Skinner seek to modify behavior by changing the contingencies under which it occurs (O'Leary and Wilson, 1975). The circle of scientifically based psychotherapies is closed by cognitive behavior therapies, which view cognitions as obeying the same laws and behavior (Meichenbaum, 1977).

In recent years, a group of therapies that are based on a concept of human nature radically different from the scientific one has gained increasing prominence. According to the humanist-existential position, the scientific view errs fundamentally in its assumption that human beings are determined. The essence of being human is the right and capacity for voluntary choice guided by purposes and values. Through our free will we can give our lives meaning despite inevitable death. The aim of therapy is to help the individual to find a purpose of life in the face of this awareness. As a consequence, the person experiences a true sense of being that enables him to integrate his physical, psychological, and spiritual natures. The goal of therapy, then, is to foster the unique human potentiality for "self-actualization" by creating optimal conditions for personal growth toward the full use of one's capacities (Maslow, 1968). Such a view holds that the essence of therapy is "the encounter," in which the therapist relates to the patient "as one existence communicating with another", or as "merging" with the patient (Havens, 1974). Through this total acceptance, the patient comes to value his own uniqueness and becomes free to exert choice and make commitments, and thus to find a meaning in life. The philosophy of existential therapy eschews specific techniques. The process of therapy is essentially an intuitive one, leading the therapist to behave differently with each of his or her patients.

Despite differences in conceptualizations and methods, which promulgators of each form of therapy emphasize, it has been difficult to show that, with a few exceptions, one form of psychotherapy is more effective than any other. At the same time, the evidence is convincing that all forms of psychotherapy produce somewhat better results than so-called spontaneous remission (Bergin and Lambert, 1978). This suggests that underneath their differences all therapies share certain components that account for much of their healing power. All involve a trusting, emotionally charged relationship between the patient and therapist, and are based on a belief system shared by both that prescribes a procedure for alleviating the patient's symptoms and disabilities. All provide opportunities for both cognitive and experiential learning with accompanying emotional arousal. All strengthen the patient's sense of mastery or self-efficacy (Bandura, 1979) by providing both explanations for the patient's difficulties and success experiences. Finally, all enable the patient to integrate through practice what has been learned (Frank, 1971).

If all forms of psychotherapy share components with significant healing effects, these components must combat a source of distress and disability that all patients coming to psychotherapy share. This may be termed "demoralization" — a state of mind characterized by degrees of hopelessness, helplessness, a sense of isolation or alienation, and a sense of worthlessness. Demoralization results when a person finds himself persistently unable to master situations that he and others expect him to handle, or when

he experiences continued distress that he cannot adequately explain.
Sometimes it is not the patient but those about him who are demoralized,
such as the families of sociopaths. Some individuals are too demoralized
to seek help, such as skid-row alcoholics, and, finally, some nondemor-
alized patients seek relief for specific symptoms, such as phobias or
compulsions, for which they have heard there is a specific treatment.
Most patients, however, seek therapy for a combination of symptoms and
demoralization (Frank, 1974).

There are three broad classes of symptoms. First, there are those
that are direct subjective manifestations of demoralization, such as anxi-
eyt, depression, and a sense of isolation. These are the most common
symptoms, and the most responsive to any form of psychotherapy. Second,
there is an equivocal group of so-called appetitive symptoms, such as
drug and alcohol abuse. These come to attention initially because they
violate social norms, but in some persons they seem to be efforts to ward
off or keep in check feelings of anxiety and despair. Finally, there are
symptom complexes that have a definable shape and course that distinguish
them from each other and from ordinary experiences and, therefore, may
deserve the term of "illness." Psychotic symptoms such as hallucinations,
delusions, and sweeping, intense mood disturbances have a significant
physiological component. In terms of current knowledge, neurotic symptoms such as phobias, compulsions, and obsessions can be most usefully
viewed either as miscarried attempts to solve internal conflicts or efforts
to gain certain gratifications from others. In any case, they tend to be
self-perpetuating and self-defeating, so that the patient becomes increasingly mired.

Whatever their source, however, symptoms interact with demoralization
in three ways. The first is that they reduce a person's coping capacity,
predisposing him to demoralizing failures. Whether the symptom be schizophrenic thought disorder, reactive depression, or an obsessional ritual,
it may cause the patient to be defeated by problems of living that asympto-
matic persons handle with ease.

Second, psychiatric symptoms, to the extent that the patient believes
them to be unique, contribute to demoralization by heightening feelings
of isolation. This accounts for one of the most powerful therapeutic features of all forms of group therapy's being "universalization" (Yalom,
1975), the discovery that others have similar symptoms and problems.

Third, all symptoms wax and wane with the degree of demoralization.
Thus, schizophrenics' thinking becomes more disorganized when they
are anxious, and obsessions and compulsions are worse when the patient
is depressed.

Most patients present themselves to therapists with specific symptoms,
and both they and their therapists believe that psychotherapy is aimed
at relieving these. I am suggesting, rather, that much of the improvement
resulting from any form of psychotherapy lies in its ability to restore the
patient's morale, with resulting diminution or disappearance of symptoms.
One must add, of course, that alleviation of the patient's symptoms may
be the best way to restore morale.

The demoralization hypothesis enables us to understand why psychotherapy is so popular today. It is because the conditions of life have
fostered widespread demoralization (Frank, 1979b; Lasch, 1978) while,
at the same time, institutions to which individuals have traditionally looked
to discover a meaning and purpose in life and to combat demoralization,
such as traditional religions, have lost much of their appeal. Psychotherapy in its protean forms has become a substitute for religion.

In contrast to the popularity of psychotherapy is a surprising lack of
solid evidence as to its effectiveness. This suggests either that the

seekers and providers of psychotherapy are suffering from a massive, shared delusion, or that the appeal of psychotherapy largely depends on characteristics that researchers do not or cannot study - that is, that cannot be evaluated by the methods of science. I am inclined to believe that the latter is nearer to the truth. There are two types of limits to the type of information that the scientific study of psychotherapy can provide (Frank, 1979a). The first are methodological and can be pushed back by improvements in describing patients and therapists and their interactions. The other class of limits, however, is more fundamental. Scientific data must be perceived by the alert, waking intellect exclusively through the senses, and the scientific method can be applied only to discrete entities existing in a time-space manifold and relating to each other by cause and effect. Countless individuals throughout history and in all cultures have reported intensely significant experiences that are not mediated by the senses, do not obey the conventional laws of causality, and cannot be fitted into the framework of time and space. Such experiences, usually termed "mystical," occasionally have more powerful healing effects than any conventional psychotherapy (Cranston, 1955; West, 1957). These healing forces, which may well subtly contribute to successful psychotherapy, will always elude the scientific method. Furthermore, despite the claim that psychotherapy is a applied science, in many ways it is closer to art and religion. It resembles religion in that it promulgates a value system that can give significance to life; it is an art in that it is a form of rhetoric, the art of persuasion (Szasz, 1978). Science cannot cast much light on religion. It can contribute to the arts, but much of their impact eludes the scientific method.

To clarify this point, let us consider another art, music. It has a scientific underpinning in the form of rules of harmony and the laws of pitch and volume, and the performer or composer must know something of these rules and facts in order to practice the art successfully. To seek to determine by scientific observation and analysis, however, whether, let us say, transactional analysis is better or worse than Gestalt therapy may be analogous to trying to use the same method to determine whether Cole Porter's music is better than Richard Rogers'. One can, to be sure, analyze their songs in terms of harmony, pitch, and volume, and create and administer any number of rating scales to cohorts of listeners; but no amount of such information will influence the individual's personal preference.

Another aspect of music that eludes scientific method is that musical ability is a gift possessed in different degrees by different people, and the quality of musical performance depends more on the musical talent of the performer than on the quality of the instrument. Anyone would much rather hear Isaac Stern playing a cheap fiddle than a novice playing a Stradivarius. Analogously, more of the effectiveness of psychotherapy may lie in ineffable, personal therapeutic qualities of the therapist than in the method he uses. Psychotherapeutic research too often studies violins when it should be studying violinists.

To the extent that psychotherapy is a combination of rhetoric and religion, its popularity has never rested on its scientifically demonstrated effectiveness; therefore, efforts to demonstrate the relative effectiveness of this or that form of psychotherapy will continue to be of more interest to researchers than to practitioners and their patients.

To come at last to the question raised by the title of this chapter, this survey leads to the conclusion that psychotherapy is certainly not dead, or even dying, but is alive and will remain so. Enough individuals benefit enough from various forms of psychotherapy to assure that they will continue to be in demand for some time to come. Evaluation of its state of health is a more difficult matter. So many variables are involved and so many changes are going on that definitive diagnosis is impossible. As I read the signs and symptoms, from the standpoint of procedures, considering the extremes first, biofeedback will probably establish a permanent, if limited, role for itself, since its instrumentation makes it appealing to certain therapists and patients and it is clearly effective for a limited spectrum of conditions. These may be more responsive to it than to other approaches.

As long as contemporary conditions of life are characterized by pervasive, continuing, and severe threats to survival and the absence of effective institutional means for counteracting the resulting demoralization, transcendental cults will probably continue to attract those who seek, and often find, serenity by surrendering themselves to groups that offer total acceptance, relieve their members of the intolerable burden of decision, and assure them of a blissful hereafter by following the teachings of a devinely inspired leader.

As self-created ways of meeting certain problems in life, self-help and consciousness raising groups will also continue to thrive.

Self-help groups and cults are supported by voluntary contributions of their members. Although cults often milk their adherents dry, they do it under the guise of religious offerings, for which their members freely make any sacrifice.

Other forms of psychotherapy charge a fee, so their future is at least indirectly linked to the state of the national economy. Participants in encounter, sensitivity, and other groups of the human potential movement pay for them out of their own pockets. One can therefore anticipate considerable falling-off of attendance along with a reduction of fees when times are bad.

The future of behavioral, cognitive, and existential psychotherapies depends to an indeterminate degree on their relative cost-benefit ratios as viewed by third-party payers, whether private or governmental. Since they assume part of the cost, their decisions will powerfully affect the future of these therapies.

Being keenly aware of this, members of the helping professions, particularly psychiatrists, psychologists, and social workers, are engaged in an intense, often bitter, struggle for the therapy insurance dollar. The battle is ostensibly being fought on high intellectual grounds as each professional group tries to define psychotherapy in such a way that it is best qualified to conduct it. Since both empirically and logically this is an impossible task, the battle is now being waged in the courts and legislatures. In the latter, the outcome will probably be determined primarily by the relative political power of the respective professions. Overall, however, as the economic shoe pinches with increasing severity, third-party payers, whether private or public, will probably define increasingly narrowly the conditions for which they will reimburse therapists, as well as limit the duration of treatment and the frequency of sessions.

These mundane, theoretically irrelevant but, unfortunately, practically crucial considerations may reduce the scope of psychotherapeutic practice, but clearly will never eliminate it. One can anticipate a drop in popularity of the more prestigious, more expensive, open-ended, long-term therapies such as psychoanalysis, simply because the results for most analysands do not justify the cost in the cold, objective judgement of third-party payers. Like existential psychotherapies, these therapies will continue to appeal to the relatively affluent, for whom they can be rewarding personal experiences.

Time-limited, sharply focused therapies, whose effectiveness can be more definitively evaluated, will probably gain relatively more support, as will group therapies. Group approaches are appealing on theoretical as well as economic grounds, since all patients are members of social networks that contribute to and are affected by the patient's symptoms.

From the standpoint of practitioners, psychiatric social workers and mental health counselors may gain at the expense of psychiatrists and psychologists, whose fees are higher.

Each therapeutic profession, however, has certain specific advantages and disadvantages with tespect to its qualifications to conduct psychotherapy with different types of patients. Psychiatrists occupy an impregnable position in treating sufferers in whom bodily disorders play an obvious, if still unclear, role. These include psychotics and patients with structural brain disease. Furthermore, since many patients have bodily as well as somatic symptoms, the psychiatrist's familiarity with bodily illness and his special social role as a healer give him a sense of security not possessed by members of other helping disciplines. This familiarity also especially qualifies psychiatrists to take the lead in the field of the psychotherapy of organic disease, an increasingly promising field as we learn more and more about the interaction of bodily and psychological states mediated by the central nervous system. Finally, psychiatrists, more than members of any other helping profession, as physicians, are thoroughly trained and indoctrinated into assuming responsibility for patients. On the other hand, medical training, by fostering an attitude of objectivity and impersonality, may be a handicap in the practice of psychotherapy, a handicap that is least likely to impede the work of psychiatric social workers, who are trained always to see patients as unique individuals. This and their greater knowledge of social stresses and supports give them an advantage for many patients. Psychologists, finally, are particularly well qualified to carry out procedures focused on the unlearning of faulty habits of behavior, thought, and feeling and the learning of more appropriate ones. They can also be expected to continue to take the lead in research pushing back the frontiers of psychotherapy.

In short, the present frenetic activity in the field of psychotherapy probably is a manifestation of hectic fever rather than robust health. The illness may be prolonged but it will not be fatal and will result in a somewhat altered appearance, including a shrinkage in size. Psychotherapy, however, will emerge with a high level of immunity against the social and economic stresses that afflict it today, and thereby will be better able to face with confidence the vicissitudes that the future may bring.

REFERENCES

Bandura, A. Self efficacy: Towards a unifying theory of behavior change. *Psychol. Rev.* 84:191-215, 1977.

Beck, A.T. *Cognitive Therapy and Emotional Disorders*. New York: International Universities Press, 1976.

Bergin, A.E. and Lambert, M.J. The evaluation of therapeutic outcomes. In *Handbood of Psychotherapy and Behavior Change:* An Empirical Analysis, S.L. Garfield and A.E. Bergin, eds. New York: John Wiley & Sons, 1978, pp. 139-189.

Cranston, R. *The Miracle of Lourdes*. New York: McGraw-Hill, 1955.

Ellis, A. *Reason and Emotion in Psychotherapy*. New York: Lyle Stuart, 1962.

Frank, J.D. Mental health in a fragmented society: The shattered crystal ball. *Amer. J. Orthopsychiat.* 33:397-408, 1979b.

Frank, J.D. The present status of outcome studies. *J. Consult. & Clin. Psychol.* 47:310-316, 1979a.

Frank, J.D. Psychotherapy: The restoration of morale. *Amer. J. Psychiat.* 131:271-274, 1974.

Frank, J.D. Therapeutic factors in psychotherapy. *Amer. J. Psychother.* 25: 350-361, 1971.

Gross, M.L. *The Psychological Society.* New York: Random House, 1978.

Havens, L.L. The existential use of the self. *Amer. J. Psychiat.* 131: 1-10, 1974.

Janov, A. *The Primal Scream: Primal Therapy, The Cure for Neurosis.* New York: Putnam, 1970.

Lasch, C. *The Culture of Narcissism: American Life in an Age of Diminishing Expectations.* New York: Norton, 1978.

Lieberman, M.A. Problems in integrating traditional group therapies with new forms. *Int. J. Group Psychother.* 27: 19-32, 1977.

Maslow, A. *Toward a Psychology of Being,* 2nd ed. New York: Harper & Row, 1968.

Meichenbaum, D. (ed.). *Cognitive Behavior Modification: An Integrative Approach.* New York: Plenum Press, 1977.

O'Leary, K.D. and Wilson, G.T. *Behavior Therapy: Application and Outcome.* Englewood Cliffs, N.J.: Prentice-Hall, 1975.

Szasz, T.S. *The Myth of Psychotherapy.* New York: Doubleday, 1978.

West, D. *Eleven Lourdes Miracles.* London: Gerald Duckworth & Co., Ltd., 1957.

Wolberg, L.R. *The Technique of Psychotherapy,* 3rd ed. New York: Grune & Stratton, 1977.

Wolpe, J. and Lazarus, A.A. *Behavior Therapy Techniques: A Guide to the Treatment of Neuroses.* New York: Pergamon Press, 1966.

Yalom, I.D. *The Theory and Practice of Group Psychotherapy,* 2nd ed. New York: Basic Books, Inc., 1975.

8

Psychiatry and Medicine: Marriage or Divorce?

William L. Webb, Jr.
Neil B. Edwards

Moore has described the relationship between psychiatry and medicine as a "long and stormy courtship with many broken engagements, an occasional annulment and sometimes outright divorce" (Moore, 1978). The analogy between psychiatry and medicine and a marriage is apt. In a marriage, two individuals with distinct identities form a union and establish ties, geographical proximity (sharing of territory), and, hopefully, mutually satisfying goals. Usually the two parties initially share a common heritage but also some distinct differences in personality and approach. The process of marriage involves growth and change. When things proceed well, there is evolution of a newly shared identity and both parties grow and develop new facets of their personalities.

Both parties, however, maintain their individual differences and specialized interests. When these differences stimulate contempt or alienation, trouble brews, and the prospect of "going one's separate way" assumes an appealing glow. Such obstacles to growth are likely to occur when an uneven balance develops in the relationship. Uneven balances occur when one partner is going through some change in identity or when external forces create unusual stress for the marriage. Medicine and psychiatry are clearly married. However, many forces, current and past, have put the union through serious tests. This chapter will explore some of the tensions, present and past, in the relationship and will advance some prognostications about the future.

A HISTORICAL PERSPECTIVE

Psychiatry and medicine share the common heritage of physicianhood. The development of psychiatry is rooted in the history of medicine. Beginning with Hippocrates, physicians have argued that insanity is an illness manifested by disordered behavior rather than somatic symptoms. As pointed out by Kety, the humanistic efforts of Pinel were based on his conviction that the inmates of the Bicetre were suffering a mental illness (Kety, 1974). The science of psychiatry is based on careful history taking and meticulous observation. From the works of physicians such as Kraepelin, Falret, and Esquirol came the basic classifications of mental illness that remain the cornerstone of our current diagnostic system.

However, with the emphatic support of the mind-body dichotomy by Descartes in the 17th century, the paths of medicine and psychiatry began to diverge. The separation of mind and body allowed the scientific study of the biological systems of the body to proceed. The development

73

of medicine hinged upon the application of the scientific method to biological systems and the in-depth study of the components of these systems.
With the information explosion in medicine following World War II, the path
along reductionism and technology has escalated.

The emphasis in psychiatry has followed another direction. The biomedical approach in psychiatry produced only an occasional breakthrough,
such as the discovery of the cause of general paresis. Empirical treatments were introduced; some effective, many ineffective, and some frankly
harmful. The basic tradition of psychiatry was founded in a humanitarian
attitude toward the mentally deranged.

With the introduction and growth of psychoanalysis, particularly in
the United States, there was a shift away from interest in the biomedical
origins of mental illness to an emphasis on psychological mechanisms underlying disordered behavior and developmental problems in the patient's
past environment. Psychoanalysis exerted a major impact and influence
on the practice of psychiatry for 20 years following the Second World War.
At a theoretical level, psychoanalysis attempted to explain psychological
phenomena in biological terms, but its practical impact was to remove psychiatry from medicine and to project the image of the psychiatrist publicly
and within the medical profession as principally a psychotherapist. The
couch replaced the stethoscope. Psychoanalysis developed its own language, which was difficult to share with medical colleagues. Psychiatrists
moved out of the mainstream of medical activity, behind closed doors of
private offices.

During this very same time period, psychiatry enjoyed a remarkable
growth in numbers of practitioners and in popularity with the public.
The National Institute of Mental Health was established and provided a
steady flow of federal funding for the training of psychiatrists. The
national concern stimulated by the many cases of battlefield neurosis in
World War II and those considered unfit for military duty because of
psychological difficulties created a new wave of interest in mental health
in the United States. However, the quality of psychiatric practice in the
1950s brought critical comment from our European colleagues. Sheppard
described American psychiatry in 1957 as follows: "There is a distaste
for detailed knowledge dismissed as 'descriptive psychiatry', antagonism
for many of the facts and concepts associated with the study of heredity,
neglect of much biological investigation, and, as Kramer has so strikingly
shown in many centers, a biased ignorance of the evolution and historical
roots in modern psychiatry" (cited in Murray, 1979). The marital state of
medicine and psychiatry had progressed to a polite and courteous separation.
The two disciplines were practiced in separate institutions. Departments
of psychiatry were established in medical schools but were regarded with
suspicion and disdain by the rest of the medical academic community.
Psychiatry's eyes were turned away from medicine to greater horizons
such as social problems, correction of human vices, and mental health for
all.

All the while, forces were at play that kept the two partners in contact and flirting with each other. The advent of the psychosomatic movement following World War II offered great promise that psychodynamic
formulations and personality profiles would assist in understanding a number of chronic illnesses known to be influenced by emotions. As Hackett
put it, there was "little practical yield from the psychosomatic theorizing
of the 30s and 40s" (Hackett, 1977), but the establishment of consultation
liaison programs in departments of psychiatry created a pathway by which
psychiatry could move back into the mainstream of the medical practice.

Other developments were also steering psychiatry back to medicine.
In the mid 1950s, the introduction of reserpine and then chlorpromazine

offered the first definitive treatment for the symptoms of psychosis.
Within a short period of time, tricyclic antidepressants made their appearance and were a major step in the control of depressive symptomatology.
The advent of effective chemotherapy that would control the severe symptomatology of psychosis had a profound effect on the practice of psychiatry.
It was possible to move the psychiatric in-patient service into the general
hospital, and this occurred with alacrity during the 1960s. Short-term
hospitalization became a reality, and it was possible to return more psychiatric patients to the community.

Then, in 1963, President Kennedy recommended passage of legislation
for the establishment of comprehensive community mental health centers.
Psychiatry shifted its focus from the medical establishment to the community. It was a heady time for American psychiatry and for the United
States. The nation, progressively involved in a conflict that threatened
the very basis of its ideals, went through a period of violent re-examin-
ation. Traditions were overturned, values were considered obsolete, and
new perspectives were the order of the day. Psychiatry, always sensitive
to the social milieu in which it exists, responded with the same kind of
turbulence and extended its pronouncements to the age-old problems of
mankind — poverty, politics, and prejudice. Some psychiatrists became
more fascinated with political activism than the practice of their profession.
The traditional authoritative roles in the medical hierarchy were replaced
with a kind of egalitarian comradery. The multidisciplinary team and therapeutic milieu gave near equal therapeutic responsibility to the well- and
not-so-well-trained. Psychiatry, by this time grossly overextended and
"madly riding off in all directions" (Hall et al., 1979), began to lose its
credibility. The radical fringe characterized psychiatry as a tool of
authority herding the socially deviant away from the public. The very
foundations of psychiatric practice were questioned. Mental illness was
declared a myth, and psychosis was characterized as a creative response
to a sick society. Psychiatry committed its most serious breach with medicine — the abolishment of the medical internship as a requirement for training in psychiatry. Experimentation in educational programs created new
tracks that de-emphasized experience in medicine for those medical students committed to psychiatry. A program was established for the creation
of a new mental health professional, the doctor of mental health. The
medical exposure in the training of the doctor of mental health was per-
functory. The marriage of psychiatry and medicine was in serious
jeopardy.

The mood of psychiatry in the 1970s and early 1980s has been
more conservative. There is a new realism, a pulling back, a retrench-
ment from overextension. Psychiatry is reflective and thoughtful about
its identity. Like a late adolescent, it takes account of its limitations,
looks at its assets, and raises questions about the future. The rapid
changes in the field and the changes in the times have produced an
identity crisis in psychiatry. It seems paradoxical that at the very
moment when psychiatry entered a new era of scientific advance —
including systematic diagnosis, evaluation, and documentation of treatment,
and a better understanding of the neurochemical substructure of
brain function — the profession should feel such insecurity.

PSYCHIATRY'S IDENTITY CRISES —ARE WE REAL DOCTORS?

The conservative mood of psychiatry matched the conservative attitude
of post-Vietnam America. Faced with serious energy problems, limited
resources, and double digit inflation, the country has, by necessity, assumed a more realistic stance. Adaptation to the environment, careful

management, accountability, and conservation of resources characterized America's attitude during the mid and late 1970s.

A central theme in psychiatry's self examination is its relationship to medicine. Some consider this a retreat to the protective umbrella of the medical establishment. Beset with competition from other mental health professionals, most notably in the area of psychotherapy, psychiatry pulls out the medical banner and dons a white coat. Others view the medical expertise and increased interest in biological systems as directly germane to the future progress of psychiatry as a medical specialty. The dimensions of the identity crisis include conceptual controversies, political and economic pressures, and the definition of the psychiatrist's future role.

CONCEPTUAL CONFLICTS, OR THE WAR OF MODELS

One of the conceptual banners carried in psychiatry's identity conflict is titled the "medical model." The medical model of mental illness has been artificially defined by its critics as a narrow, largely biological, linear view of mental illness. Caricatured in the extreme, it is said to hold that a twisted thought represents a twisted molecule. Critics of the medical model have complained that it is too mechanistic and pseudoscientific, or have stated outright that mental illness is a myth. Szasz states that mental illness is a myth whose function is to disguise the bitter pill of moral conflicts in human relations (Yasher, 1974). Laing maintains that we live in a sick and corrupt society, and that the psychotic experience represents a creative response to that sick environment (Laing, 1971).

Closely aligned to the myth concept is the challenge to psychiatric diagnosis most frequently called "labeling theory" (Eisenberg, 1977). Labeling theory maintains that psychiatric diagnosis has no validity and is but a convenient way to identify deviants for the purpose of restricting their freedom and removing them from society. The labeling theory reached its peak when a group under the direction of D. L. Rosenhan deliberately set about to simulate psychosis and were hospitalized, diagnosed, treated, and discharged from a state hospital (Rosenhan, 1973). Kety points out that Rosenhan's trick in no way supported his faulty conclusion that psychiatric diagnosis cannot "tell sanity from insanity," but was a simple exercise in the stimulation of illness (Kety, 1974). This is something that is easily replicated by patients who produce factitious illness to gain entrance to general medical hospitals where they may receive diagnostic studies and treatment.

Kety, a staunch defender of the medical approach to mental illness, states, "The medical model is an evolving intellectual process involving observation, description, differentiation, and research. It moves from a recognition and palliation of symptoms to specific etiology, pathogenesis, and treatment." Further, "the medical model is an excellent example of the application of the scientific method to human suffering" (Kety, 1974). Ludwig and Othmer, on the other hand, take a rather extreme view — that when no biological dysfunction can be demonstrated or presumed (in mental illness) no disease exists. They suggest that psychiatrists abrogate their responsibility as doctors by treating the non-sick (Ludwig and Othmer, 1977). Weiner has thoroughly examined four types of medical model: the infectious, cellular pathology, diagnostic, and curative. He points out that biological systems are highly complex. The models used to explain these systems are neither linear nor simple (Weiner, 1978).

All agree that every disease has social and psychological consequences, and Engel calls for a new model for all of medicine based on the systems approach that takes account of biological, psychological, and social vari-

ables in the evolution of the disease process (Engel, 1977).
Bursten voices the suspicion that all the talk about medical models is
largely rhetoric, motivated by economic pressures, political concerns,
and the status of technology and hard data in modern medicine (Bursten,
1979). He states that, since models are simply belief systems to make
easier the understanding of complex theoretical propositions, psychiatry
should maintain maximal conceptual freedom. He suggests that the specialty of psychiatry may require a very wide conceptual base to encompass
the task of weaving complex systems into a holistic understanding.

IS PSYCHIATRY AN ENDANGERED SPECIES?
PROBABLY NOT – JUST WELL REGULATED

From early times, psychiatry has dealt with large segments of society
who are without advocates and who have become the responsibility of
public institutions. The organizers of the American Psychiatric Association were the superintendents of state hospitals. In recent years, psychiatry has been accused of running away from the public sector, but
surveys reveal that 43 percent of psychiatrists are still involved in some
form of public service (Brown, 1976). The association of psychiatry with
state hospitals has done little to improve the public or self-image of the
profession. The chronic underfunding of these state institutions by state
and federal governments has made them the constant victim of class action
suits and exposés in the media, and the subject matter of best-selling
novels and movies. None of these portrays the profession in a favorable
light.
The influx of foreign medical graduates into vacant positions in the
state hospital system established a two-class system of care (Mittel, 1977).
The well-staffed private, often university-affiliated, hospitals with largely
American-trained psychiatrists, and the poorly staffed, largely unaffiliated
state hospitals with foreign medical graduates provided a sharp contrast.
The number of training programs proliferated in state hospitals and, at
one point, one third of the trainees in American psychiatry were foreign
medical graduates, mainly in state hospital training programs.
The advent of the community mental health center programs created
greater insecurities for psychiatrists. The community mental health
movement stressed the team approach. The influx of other mental health
professionals to meet the mass of service demands has markedly diluted
the influence and prestige of the psychiatrists in the community mental
health movement (Glickman, 1979). Psychiatry has felt aggressive competition from psychology and social work. This reached a new peak four
years ago, when the American Psychological Association filed a suit with
the Federal Trade Commission to grant psychologists admitting privileges
to general hospital psychiatric in-patient units and medical responsibilities
on those services. A recent survey revealed that a sizable number of
people do not know the difference between a psychologist and a psychiatrist (Clarke and Martin, 1978).
The new relationship with other mental health professionals has been
very difficult for many psychiatrists. Either stretched very thin as
"supervisors" or "team leaders" exerting tenuous control over a number of
mental health workers, or reduced to the ignominious role of prescription
signers, psychiatrists have fled the mental health centers. The community
mental health movement has steadily come under the influence of psychologists and social workers. Paradoxically, psychiatrists in mental health
centers have been forced into functioning more as primary care physicians,
taking histories, performing physicals, and keeping a watchful eye for
the possibility of undetected medical complications (Munoz, 1978; Finerao,

1978). However, in many circumstances, psychiatrists have functioned largely as administrators, and their responsibilities, economic and political, are far removed from their medical training.

The community mental health movement, based largely on declining federal support, has suffered the same fate as state hospitals. There is inadequate support to establish the total aftercare system necessary to meet the needs of the chronic psychotic population. The crowding of patients into community nursing homes and inadequate supervision of chronic psychotics in the community have reflected poorly on the community mental health movement, and many lay this at the door of psychiatry.

In the early 1970s, the love affair between psychiatry and the federal government began to cool. Federal support for training in psychiatry, plentiful in the 1960s, has been steadily cut back. The federal government, feeling that the rise in the numbers of psychiatrists from 4,700 in 1947 to 32,000 in 1979 provided an adequate boost to the profession, shifted support to the training of primary care physicians (Eaton, 1980). Although recent efforts to get psychiatry declared a shortage specialty have been moderately successful, the profession will never enjoy the support that it received in the past from the federal government, and will very likely be subject to regulation, as are other specialties, with respect to the total number and geographic distribution of future psychiatrists.

None of the national health insurance proposals to date includes support for mental illness as part of the package. Insurance companies have become skeptical about reimbursement for psychiatric care. Although repeated studies have demonstrated that third-party coverage for psychiatric care is not abused, there is still the concern that comprehensive insurance for mental illness would be an incentive for people to seek unnecessary help for emotional difficulties and, thus, escalate costs. This same suspiciousness characterizes the review of claims for psychiatric treatment. Claims for mental treatment are more carefully scrutinized and are frequently reviewed by claims boards. It is clear that future psychiatric practice will be characterized by very careful peer review and frequent chart audits as the profession comes under greater regulation by the government and other third-party carriers. Incentives will undoubtedly be introduced to correct the maldistribution of psychiatrists and to further extend mental health coverage to underserved populations — children, the poor, and the aged (Sumers, 1977). Psychiatrists still tend to cluster in cities on the East and West Coasts. Forty percent of medical care is currently government supported, and that will doubtlessly increase. Some feel that national health insurance will push medicine and psychiatry closer together, while others fear that psychiatry is truly endangered.

Psychiatric education reflects some of psychiatry's identity problems. Recruitment of medical students into psychiatric residency programs has dropped from 12 percent in the years following World War II to 3.4 percent in 1978 (Eaton, 1980). Surveys reveal that psychiatry still holds a low status with many medical students. Despite the breakthroughs in psychopharmacology and neurochemical understanding of brain functions, many students still feel psychiatry is vague and that the profession is at war with itself. It is clear that the current 238 programs in adult and child psychiatry are too many. With a sharp cutback in the number of available foreign medical graduates, many of these programs will die of attrition.

WILL THE FUTURE PSYCHIATRIST BE A "REAL DOCTOR"?

Many anecdotes attest to the anxiety psychiatrists feel about whether or not they are genuine medical doctors. Hackett has remarked, "If we are not at home in medicine, we are homeless" (Hackett, 1977). This anxiety is not lessened when those in community mental health state that the future of psychiatry lies in managing systems and providing backup support to other frontline mental health professionals. What will the future relationship of psychiatry and medicine be?

Our guess is that psychiatry, which traditionally has cared for the mentally ill, will continue its medical orientation in the future. As Kety puts it, "The psychiatrist is best equipped to carry out responsibilities toward the mentally ill on the basis of a broad background in medicine, clinical psychology, and the scientific method" (Kety, 1974); or, put another way by Eaton, "The psychiatrist specializes in disordered behavior which is the final common pathway of biology, psychology, and sociology" (Eaton, 1980).

Whatever additional expertise the psychiatrist may acquire, managerial or consultation skills, the core responsibility of psychiatry lies now, and will continue to reside, in the care of the individual patient (Hill, 1978). Essential to this task is the special integrity of the doctor-patient relationship. As Ludwig and Othmer point out, such a relationship entails awesome responsibility and access to specialized information, and is accompanied by serious ethical constraints (Ludwig and Othmer, 1977). This relationship is forged in the medical tradition of responsibility for life and limb and demands a high level of emotional maturity.

Will psychiatry abandon psychotherapy? This seems highly unlikely. Practicing psychotherapy is in no way inconsistent with one's medical responsibilities. Many primary care physicians will be practicing psychotherapy as part of their management of patients with chronic medical illness. An essential appeal of psychiatry is its emphasis on the exciting and emotionally rewarding interactions of psychotherapy. The range of therapies is broadening and is increasingly involving couples, families, and groups. Psychiatry's future does not lie in artifically barring itself from these developments. Recent studies show that psychotherapy, exclusively or in combination with drugs, is the treatment modality of choice in certain emotional disorders such as reactive depression (Hall, 1980). We can expect competition, and ultimately the question of who does psychotherapy will be established in the marketplace.

Psychiatry today and tomorrow places greater responsibility on the individual practitioner for general medical knowledge. Some have attempted to delineate areas of special expertise for psychiatrists, such as medical emergencies, drug interactions, or basic medical treatment for common ailments; but such delineations are clearly too limited. The cornerstone of psychiatric practice today and tomorrow will be differential diagnosis. The emphasis in DSM-III on diagnosis by inclusion and exclusion criteria demonstrates the importance of systematic diagnosis in future practice. The implementation of differential diagnosis requires a working knowledge of medicine. It must exceed that of a physician's assistant. A recent study by Hall and others (1980) revealed that 46 percent of chronically mentally ill patients had undetected medical illnesses, one half of which had a direct bearing on the disordered behavior manifested by the patient.

A number of authors have called for greater scientific knowledge and more research into mental illness in the future (Guze, 1977). Greenhill outlines the need for a "clinical science of psychiatry" (Greenhill, 1978). The medical approach of symptom recognition, symptom clustering in the evolution of syndromes, and the identification of subtypes by biological or psychological means is the ideal application of science in the care of the mentally ill. The 1970s have seen America become the world center for the study of psychiatric genetics. There have been major advances in psychoendocrinology and the neurochemical basis of brain function. As we become more scientific, we are likely to become more medical.

The future of psychiatry hinges on the resiliency and flexibility of the young psychiatrist of tomorrow. To us this means maximum conceptual freedom. Psychiatry's major contribution to medicine, past and future, is a broader conception of the patient and his problem, which provides new understandings and insights into both diagnosis and treatment. Whenever psychiatry has backed itself into a rigid conceptual corner, it has reaped the consequences. Our future may indeed be uncertain should this happen again.

MAKING IT WITH MEDICINE

The establishment of psychiatric consultation liaison programs in several major teaching centers in the late 1940s and early 1950s has been important in bringing the two specialties together. Internists trained in programs where the relationship was strong and genuine bear the imprint of that training. In those centers where they have established academic leadership, they continue a tradition of sincere interest in the whole patient, not just his biological functioning. All who have worked in consultation liaison psychiatry attest to the ambivalence that exist between the psychiatrist and his fellow medical colleagues. Some have likened medicine's protestations of interest in the psychosocial dimensions of patient care to motherhood and apple pie — American myths that are seldom genuinely realized (McKegney, 1977). The psychiatrist frequently settles for the quick patient-oriented consultation or simply takes the patient off the hands of the medical service. The quick consultation seldom achieves the goals of a true liaison relationship, where ongoing communication with the medical and nursing staff exerts a critically beneficial impact on patient care.

Most liaison activities, until recent years, were oriented around medical and surgical in-patient services. Most of the literature is concerned with these experiences. Only recently have liaison activities with out-patient populations been reported. Psychiatry's efforts with family practice residency programs that emphasize ambulatory care have been quite variable (Fisher, 1978). In a number of training sites, family practice programs have rejected psychiatric input and have set about extablishing their own divisions of behavioral science. Psychiatry has again felt the competition of the "medical" psychologists who, with internists and family physicians, are developing the new specialty of behavioral medicine.

The development of these competitive liaisons is symptomatic of medicine's increasing awareness that it is not making it with the public. The image of the doctor as he surrounds himself with a proliferating technology, has become increasingly remote from the patient. Americans are feeling that something is wrong and missing in their contacts with medicine. Medical costs continue to rise, but you can't get a doctor to do a home visit. Psychiatry has an important role in reintroducing the human factor into medicine — if we don't get beat out by the psychologists. Medicine is oriented toward tests and techniques to the extreme. The behavioral paradigms offered by the psychologists have a compelling simplicity. Psychologists, schooled in an academic experimental tradition, and armed with computers and paper-pencil tests, offer a much more tempting "certainty" than the conceptual generalities espoused by the psychiatrist. It is tempting to jump to the conclusion that psychiatry has a natural bridging function because it involves training in two disciplines — medicine and psychology; but, in truth, many psychiatrists are not very well trained in psychology *or* medicine. Their dynamic formulations and vague references to systems theory are pale by comparison to well-trained experimental psychologists who know how to handle data, are knowledgeable about group process, and know how to be persuasive. Most of what modern psychologists know is well worth psychiatry's knowing. We must incorporate their knowledge to broaden our spectrum of therapeutic effectiveness and to sharpen our communication with medicine.

Does psychiatry have a viable home in medicine, or are we in the same league with the player piano? Every evidence points to medicine's need for psychiatry and vice versa. Conservative estimates report the prevalence of significant emotional difficulties in medical populations at somewhere between 40 and 70 percent (McKegney, 1977).

Depression or misery would appear to be the most common emotional affliction in the medically ill (Hall et al., 1979). How much depression seen in medical illness is reactive and secondary, and how much represents true primary affective disorder, remains to be clarified. What is apparent is that patients with bona fide undiagnosed primary affective disorder most often visit their doctor for "medical" complaints. The majority are not diagnosed or are misdiagnosed as having anxiety problems and are treated with benzodiazepines that worsen the depressive symptomatology (Weisman, personal communication). Psychiatrists know how to diagnose and treat depressive disorders very effectively.

Depressive disorders commonly simulate medical illness, and a change in the affective state can be the first sign of underlying organic disease (Hall et al., 1979). The differential diagnosis of this common medical problem can be accomplished only by someone who is truly knowledgeable about psychiatric diagnosis and medical problems. At present, this can be accomplished only by a well-trained psychiatrist.

The steady increase in the number and variety of psychotropic medications requires a physician who knows their side effects and how to consult with his medical colleagues concerning the use of these agents in the elderly and the medically ill. Most internists have only a superficial acquaintance with the psychotropic medications and may thus use them inappropriately or in inadequate dosage. The increased technology of modern medicine has brought with it a host of emotional problems. Intensive care, burn, and dialysis units require constant consultation to reduce psychological morbidity. The prevalence of psychotic reactions and suicidal depressions in specialized units can be markedly reduced by enlightened psychiatric consultation.

Medicine's success with acute illnesses has produced an over-representation of chronic conditions in modern medical practice. Patients are living longer, into the sixth and seventh decades. Aging is associated with the rapid increase in emotional disturbances and disordered behavior. Psychiatry has an important role in the care of the elderly and chronically ill.

Recently, it has been appreciated that the principal disability associated with chronic benign pain is abnormal illness behavior that builds up around the chronic condition. Abnormal illness behavior becomes the important treatment objective. Psychiatry is participating actively in the interdisciplinary approach to the diagnosis and management of chronic pain (Hall et al., 1979).

Despite the development of the most advanced medical treatment technology in the world, American medicine has still not had a significant impact on the health of the nation. Health is a highly individual matter. It relates directly to the life-style of the individual, his values and habits. Medicine is constantly losing the battle of influencing people into habits that produce good health. It has been estimated that the majority of patients fail to comply with the doctor's recommendations. Patients are particularly resistant to changes in habits or life-style, and at least 50 percent are not compliant in taking their medications. In many instances, this failure to comply has serious health consequences. Psychiatry should be in the forefront of research that develops better methods for increasing patient compliance and reducing risk factors by effecting strategic changes in the patient's life-style and/or habits.

Engel has made the point well that the biomedical model, so long the forefront of medical advance, is no longer adequate to modern medical practice (Engel, 1977). He calls for a biopsychosocial model that takes account of how biological, social, and psychological systems interact to produce states of health and disease. It is apparent that life changes have profound effects upon the onset and course of disease. Psychiatry can seize the initiative in leading medicine to this new conceptual framework. We must have a well-developed clinical science that elucidates the mechanisms by which social and psychological systems exert influences on the biological systems and how this feeds back into the individual patient's behavior and mind-set. The biopsychosocial conceptual framework for the practice of medicine offers the ideal to which good marriages aspire — a true union.

REFERENCES

Bursten, B. Psychiatry and the rhetoric of models. *Am. J. Psychiat.* 136(5):661-666, 1979.

Brown, B. The life of psychiatry. *Am. J. Psychiat.* 133(5):489-493, 1976.

Clarke, R. and Martin, G. The image of psychiatry today. *Psychiat. Opin.* 15(11):10-16, 1978.

Eaton, J.S. Psychiatrist and psychiatric education. In *Comprehensive Textbook of Psychiatry*, 3rd ed., A.M. Freedman, and H.I. Kaplan (eds). Baltimore: Williams & Wilkins Co., in press (1980).

Eisenberg, L. Psychiatry and society. *N. Engl. J. Med.* 296(16):903-910, 1977.

Engel, G.L. The need for a new medical model — a challenge for biomedicine. *Science* 196(4286):129-135, 1977.

Finerao, A.D. The medical psychiatrist as primary care physician. *Psychiat. Opin.* 15(5):17-21, 1978.

Fisher, J.V. What the family physician expects from the psychiatrist. *Psychosomatics* 19(9):523-527, 1978.

Glickman, L. The continuing demedicalization of psychiatry. *Psychiat. Opin.* 16(5):15-21, 1979.

Greenhill, M. Toward a theory of clinical science. *Psychosomat.* 19(9):519-520, 1978.

Guze, S. The future of psychiatry: Medicine or social science. *J. Nerv. Ment. Dis.* 165(4):225-230, 1977.

Hackett, T. The psychiatrist: In the mainstream or on the banks of medicine? *Am. J. Psychiat.* 134(4):432-434, 1977.

Hall, R.C.W. Depression. In *Physicial Illness Presenting as Psychiatric Disease*. New York: Spectrum Publications, Inc., in press (1980).

Hall, R.C.W.; Gardner, E.R.; Stickney, S.; LeCann, A.F.; Perl, M. Physical illness presenting as psychiatric disease II: Analysis of a state hospital population. *Arch. Gen. Psychiat.*, in press (1980).

Hall, R.C.W., Perl, M., DeVaul, R., Stickney, S.K., Faillace, L.A., Hall, A.K. A comparison of tricyclic antidepressants and analgesics in the management of chronic postoperative surgical pain. Presented at the 26th Annual Meeting, Academy of Psychosomatic Medicine, San Francisco, California, October, 1979.

Hill, D. The qualities of a good psychiatrist. *Brit. J. Psychiat.* 133:97-105, 1978.

Kety, S. From rationalization to reason. *Am. J. Psychiat.* 131(9):957-963, 1974.

Laing, R.D. *Sanity, Madness and the Family,* 2nd ed. New York: Basic Books, 1971.

Ludwig, A. and Othmer, E. The medical basis of psychiatry. *Am. J. Psychiat.* 134(10):1087-1092, 1977.

McKegney, P. Psychiatry and primary care — a need for problem solving. *Psychiat. Opin.* 14:1, 1977.

Mittel, N. The foreign medical graduate in American psychiatry

Moore, G. The adult psychiatrist in the medical environment. *Am. J. Psychiat.* 135(4):413-419, 1978.

Munoz, R. The psychiatrist as a primary physician. *Psychiat. Opin.* 15(5):14-16, 1978.

Murray, R.M. A reappraisal of American psychiatry. *Lancet.* 1:255-258, 1979.

Rosenhan, D.L. On being sane in insane places. *Science* 179:250-258, 1973.

Sumers, A.R. Accountability, public policy, and psychiatry. *Am. J. Psychiat.* 134(9):959-965, 1977.

Weiner, H. The illusion of simplicity: The medical model revisited. *Am. J. Psychiat.* 135 (Jy Supp):22-27, 1978.

Yasher, S. The outspoken Dr. Szasz, controversial foe of involuntary psychiatry. *Mod. Med.* 1974.

9

Credibility: The Problem with Psychiatry's Return to Medicine

Michael K. Popkin
Thomas B. Mackenzie

> *Moreover, tell me this truly, that I may surely know, who
> are thou and whence of the sons of men? Where is thy city
> and where are they that begat thee? Where now is thy
> swift ship moored, that brought thee thither with thy god-
> like company? Hast thou come as a passenger on another's
> ship, while they set thee ashore and went away?*
>
> — *The Odyssey*, Homer

Amidst the current tumult and shouting there is frequently heard the
rallying cry that psychiatry's course must be steered back to medicine.
Hackett (1977) carefully delineated the saga of psychiatry's progressive
estrangement from general medicine. He offered guidelines for psychiatry's survival and re-entry from the "banks of medicine" into the "mainstream". Likewise, Hall, Faillace, and Perl (1979) enumerated specific
remedies for psychiatry's present plight; these included special emphasis
on the re-establishment of ties with organized medicine. But can a *uni-
laterally* desired reconciliation involving psychiatry's proposed return to
the medical model be readily achieved? Or has the medicine-psychiatry
dyad been irrevocably altered by the protracted separation? Like
Odysseus, what can psychiatry expect as it returns from years of wander-
ing, fighting the "Cyclops" of community mental health, the Sirens of
many causes, and other assorted trials? (For example, Is medicine as
constant as Penelope?)

The arguments for the reassertion of psychiatry's medical identity are
varied. Two appear particularly meaningful. First, it is training in medicine that distinguishes the psychiatrist from others in the mental health
arena. To forego the physician's mantle is to honor the suggestion that
psychiatry offers no skills beyond those of psychology, social work,
and other mental health disciplines. Second, the exponential advances of
biological psychiatry can be expected to necessitate in their clinical application a thorough grounding in medicine. By way of example, consider
the knowledge currently required for responsible use of lithium carbonate
or any tricyclic antidepressant. Yet such arguments speak only to psychiatry's perspective of a proposed re-entry. Half the equation stands
strangely absent. How might medicine view this prospect? Has it been
assumed that psychiatry, one true identity is revealed and proved, will
be welcomed home? If this is an underlying assumption in the call for re-
entry, its merits may be questionable.

At present, psychiatry's banner vis a vis medicine is principally carried by its consultation-liaison endeavor. Consideration of the consultation experience and medicine's receptivity to it is in order. This might be expected to clarify the feasibility of a proposed return and offer indication if this should be hastened or tempered. Fundamental to this step is an examination of the medical credibility and privilege extended to psychiatry in the consultation-liaison context. This sheds *surprising* light upon medicine's vantage point. The information from this vanguard area may at present be the solitary contribution to weighing the proposed course at a crucial juncture.

Despite the proliferation of consultation-liaison services in the 1970s, there is clear evidence that such services remain rampantly *underutilized* in the general hospital setting. As Koran and his associates have noted, the prevalence of psychiatric disorders (20 to 50 percent) greatly exceeds the psychiatric referral rate (0.5 to 10 percent) (Koran, et al., 1979). In response to these discouraging observations, proponents of the return to medicine movement are likely to emphasize the liaison function of C-L activities. They might counter that underutilization reflects the extent of the need for the informal education and attitudinal change regarded as the central thrust of liaison. To date, this sort of rhetoric must be regarded as speculative and unproved. Yet objective data regarding psychiatry's medical credibility in the consultation context does exist.

In an effort to characterize the effectiveness of consultative activities, we have initiated development of a Consultation-Liaison Outcome Evaluation System (CLOES). In the initial phase of this work, consultees' responses to psychiatric consultation have been quantified in three areas: recommendations for drugs, recommendations for diagnostic action, and representation of consultants' psychiatric diagnoses. Proceeding from retrospective review of medical records, the work has utilized specific quantitative criteria to rate consultees' responses as either concordant (C), partially concordant (PC), or nonconcordant (NC). Variables critical to the respective outcomes have likewise been identified.

In a series of 200 consecutive consultations performed by a teaching service in a university hospital setting, 68 percent of all psychotropic recommendations resulted in physician responses rated C, and 24 percent, NC (Popkin, et al., 1979). Responses did not differ according to drug group (e.g., tricyclic antidepressant, major tranquilizer, or minor tranquilizer) but did vary according to category of recommendation (e.g., start, adjust, continue, discontinue). Lowest concordant rates (about 60 percent) were observed with recommendations to start or to discontinue psychotropic medication (Popkin, et al., 1980). The basis for this observation may reflect aversion on the part of consultees to more radical clinical actions. Alternatively, the directives to start or stop a psychotropic may be perceived by consultees as a criticism of their clinical judgment and an affront to their narcissism. In either case, the overall concordance rate, approaching 70 percent, appears encouraging. An optimal concordance rate remains to be established; 100 percent concordance would likely reflect indiscriminate or unthinking adherence. Therefore, the observed drug concordance rate of about 70 percent indicates that, in the context of drug management, the psychiatric consultant is extended considerable medical credibility and privilege. Cross-disciplinary comparative studies now completed by our group substantiate this finding (Popkin, et al., in press).

A similar investigation of consultees' concordance with psychiatric consultants' recommendations for diagnostic action found only 53 percent of responses rated C (Popkin, Mackenzie, and Callies, 1980). Of note, consultees' responses were independent of the specific action advised:

additional consultation, psychological test, diagnostic procedure, or laboratory determination. Concordance was shown to be a function of the age of the patient, the resultant psychiatric diagnosis, and the length of hospitalization. The 53 percent concordance rate, independent of consultee service, must be considered a disturbing result. Why should recommendations for diagnostic action, when made by a psychiatric consultant, lead to nearly a 50 percent nonconcordance rate?

Observing that concordance with diagnostic recommendations rose to 84 percent when the patient was diagnosed by the consultant as having organic mental disorder, we have previously argued that consultees are inclined to view patients referred for psychiatric consultation from a simplistic functional-organic dichotomy. "Once the functional category has been invoked to account for psychiatric features, consultees appear to consider medical aspects and approaches concluded. Thus the designation "functional" may be equated with a nonmedical entity by consultees. The psychiatric consultant may then be beckoned as an intermediary, buffer, or resource person with regard to disposition, but *HARDLY AS A FELLOW PHYSICIAN* whose province might reasonably include making recommendations for diagnostic action" (Popkin, Mackenzie, and Callies, 1980). It was concluded that, in the context of advising evaluative actions, the psychiatrist is inconsistently afforded medical credibility and privilege by consultees.

Taken together, the drug and diagnostic recommendation studies suggest that the medical credibility and identity of the psychiatric consultant as perceived by his medical colleagues cannot be safely regarded as a "given". Rather, the data suggest that there may be a wide gap to medical credibility for psychiatric consultants. This prospect is underscored by the findings in a study examining the adequacy of consultees' representations of consultants' psychiatric diagnoses (Callies, et al., 1980). Using specific outcome criteria, just 50 percent of representations were rated concordant. Of the NC cases, two thirds involved omissions and one third, inaccurate representations. The omissions speak to the likelihood that consultees perceive psychiatric diagnoses as having little utility or import. In turn, the inaccurate representations suggested a limited grasp of psychiatric nosology by consultees.

The data and the outcome studies cited here should serve to reflect that serious problems do exist with psychiatry's proposed return to medicine and the medical model. The underutilization of psychiatric expertise in the medical setting and the variable perceptions of the psychiatric consultant's medical identity cannot be ignored or go unappreciated. During psychiatry's protracted sojourn, medicine, like Penelope, has been wooed by many suitors. However, it has not found it necessary to unravel on a nightly basis its daily work. Rather, it has most certainly reconceptualized its notions of psychiatry. From our vantage point, clinical medicine without psychiatry's companionship has increasingly turned away or distanced itself from the realm of emotional and behavioral considerations. These areas and concerns may now readily be relinquished to psychiatry, but hardly from the conviction that they constitute medical entities. It must be noted that many of psychiatry's medical brethren may harbor (if not espouse) views and conceputalizations of psychiatry as a decidedly nonmedical enterprise. Such a vantage point may be the toll of the lengthy separation; at best, the rift has done little to challenge such perceptions. These prospects should sound a note of caution to those who champion the return to medicine movement.

If the vanguard consultation experience has validity for the whole of psychiatry, and if the price of long separation has been to reinforce notions of psychiatry as nonmedical, what can be counseled?

We regard two points as critical in response to the question. First, there must be recognition that, at present, medicine and psychiatry function from somewhat disparate conceptual frameworks. Any proposed recognition must begin with the effort to grasp and appreciate fully the perceptions of the other member of the dyad. We see little evidence to date of such effort on the part of psychiatry. Reunions are not unilateral phenomena, and the discipline can ill afford to ignore its proposed partner. Areas of conceptual disparity as well as concordance must be identified and addressed. For example, reliance by medicine on simplistic functional-organic dichotomies in the approach to psychatric disorder must be confronted.

Second, psychiatry will have to earn its medical credibility and privilege. For many of us, this will require more than the Odyssean stringing of the old bow.

REFERENCES

Callies, A.L., Popkin, M.K. Mackenzie, T.B., Mitchell, J. Consultees' representations of consultants' psychiatric diagnoses. *Am. J. Psychiat.* 137:1250-1253, 1980.

Hackett, T.P. The psychiatrist: In the mainstream or on the banks of medicine? *Am. J. Psychiat.* 134:432-434, 1977.

Hall, R.C.W., Faillace, L.A., Perl, M. Role diffusion and "the death of psychiatry". *Psychiat. Opin.* 16:21-23, 1979.

Koren, L.M., Van Natta, J., Stephen, J.R., Pascualy, R. Patients reactions to psychiatric consultation. *JAMA* 241:1603-1605, 1979.

Popkin, M.K., Mackenzie, T.B., Callies, A.L. Consultees' concordance with consultants' recommendations for diagnostic action. *J. Nervous Mental Dis.* 168:9-12, 1980.

Popkin, M.K., Mackenzie, T.B., Callies, A.L. and Cohn, J.N. An An interdisciplinary comparision of consultation outcomes. *Arch. Gen. Psych.* (in press).

Popkin, M.K., Mackenzie, T.B., Hall, R.C.W.. Callies, A.L. Consultees' concordance with consultants' psychotropic drug recommendations related variables. *Arch. Gen. Psych.* 37:1017-1021, 1980.

Popkin, M.K., Mackenzie, T.B., Hall, R.C.W., Garrard, J. Physicians' concordance with consultants' recommendations for psychotropic medication. *Arch. Gen. Psych.* 36:386-389, 1979.

10

Crisis in American Psychiatry

Herzl R. Spiro

No planner ever set out to design a psychiatric snakepit. So why have they emerged in virtually every century in the history of Western medicine? And by what excess of hubris do we, the erstwhile planners of the late twentieth century, conclude our brilliant plans will yield nothing but gleaming pavilions of compassionate care and lives of happy community adjustment for the chronically ill?

If it is the awareness that nonspecific effects of dignified humane environments and home care help avoid chronic institutional breakdown syndromes, our optimism is misplaced. The importance of light, air, human scale environment, and so on has been periodically rediscovered since the era of classical medicine 2,000 years ago. The buildings constructed by the practitioners of "moral therapy" became the crowded warehouses of the mid-nineteenth century. Each century's bright dream has become the next century's nightmare.

The crisis of in-patient psychiatry is that our planning may be far worse than that of our predecessors. In the absence of forceful intervention, the snakepits will be far worse by the year 2,000 than those we have heretofore seen.

THE PROBLEM

Denial of Chronicity

Some planners of the 1960s and 1970s believed that the act of removing chronic patients from hospitals and placing them in community settings would interrupt the cycle of illness. As Brill points out (Brill, 1975), "It is ironic that 100 years earlier Dorothea Dix had persuaded legislators to create these hospitals in order to prevent chronicity, because she assumed that the patient must be taken from the home and placed in a mental hospital to be cured. Within a century, the hospital and the home had traded places as cause and cure (or prevention) of chronicity in mental disorder." In the United States, the hospital population dropped from its 1955 peak census of 560,000 patients to a 1975 census of 170,000 (Meyer, 1976).

But did the base rate of illness change? The admission rate for schizophrenia has remained remarkably constant. No serious epidemiologist has even suggested that the rate of chronic illness has decreased during the 17 years of the community psychiatry revolution. Has this produced a revision of sociological theory? Has Sarbin recanted his attributions that role causes illness (Sarbin and Mancuso, 1972)? Has Scheff retracted his view that labeling produces the dysfunctions of chronicity (Scheff, 1966)? Hardly. The obvious conclusion that the natural history of untreated and chronic process schizophrenia and certain organic brain syndromes with psychosis produces states of severe disability goes ignored. The myth of mental illness (Szasz, 1963) remains popular conventional "wisdom". Severe disability is greeted with equally profound denial. Such impairment is attributed to the doctor, the venal psychiatrist, who labels his way to wealth and hospitalizes for fun and profit! Or at the least, the poor, misguided idealist who wasted years learning medical models that obviously are the cause of, not the treatment for, these disorders!

In past centuries, treatment approaches have also been built on mythical explanations. Sprenger and Kramer burnt schizophrenics as witches for the best of motives (Zilboorg, 1941). The modern Sprenger and Kramer send the descendent sisters of these patients "to the community," where they wrap themselves in newspapers for warmth and dwell in New York subway stations. So long as basic chronic illness is denied, so long as incorrect attributions of etiology dominate the popular view, so long as denial replaces reason, rational planning becomes impossible. One source of crisis in in-patient care for chronic mental illness is that planning is not based on current knowledge about chronic mental illness. Instead, plans are built on myth, pseudoscience, and blatant denial.

The Destruction of Psychiatric Hospitals

Such attitudes toward chronic mental illness hardly attract young physicians to psychiatric practice in public institutions. The medically minded will practice near general hospital units that sort out the chronically ill and within days discharge them to ... to whom? Those young psychiatrists who find psychosocial models of interest may find out-patient therapy for neurotics, self-limiting disorders, and acute depressives less stigmatizing, more lucrative, and far less harrowing.

The staffing patterns of government hospitals have always been unsatisfactory. Solomon (1958), at the outset of the current "revolution," noted that only 15 states had greater than 50 percent of the minimum staffing standards for state hospitals. With the stoppage in the flow of foreign graduates, a primary source of physicians was removed. As the percentage of American medical school graduates entering psychiatry diminishes, the supply of doctors get yet tighter. Poor staffing means unacceptable patient-doctor ratios, unacceptable patient care, and unacceptable conditions for medical practice. A vicious cycle ensues, which lead to physician resignations and still worse staffing patterns.

Not only is the quantitative supply of doctors deficient; the role of physicians has changed. The antimedical model has quietly penetrated the administrative hierarchy. One cause is self-serving beliefs by non-physicians that medical ignorance is not only acceptable but even is a necessary prerequisite to decision-making authority in the management of the mental health enterprise. Once, a chain of medical authority led from the person responsible for the individual patient, to the unit chief, to the division chief, to the hospital superintendent, to the state commissioner — all psychiatrists. Now those psychiatrists brave enough to enter state service may serve under a civil service psychologist (if they're lucky!) who, in turn, reports to an administrative bureaucrat who, in turn, channels through several more bureaucrats to a political appointee who is Secretary for [In] Human Services. By the time the occasional psychiatrist consultant has helped the instant expert learn what a patient is, chances are he will find a new political appointee in the post. It has been repeatedly demonstrated that only systems and hospitals run by psychiatrists can attract adequate psychiatric staffing. Bureaucrats more interested in power than patient care have helped create the crisis in in-patient care.

Not only is the career staff a phenomenon of the past; the physical plant has been allowed to deteriorate to a disastrous level. Few state systems have modernized facilities during the deinstitutionalization craze. Even if state and local government could be persuaded to replace decrepit hospitals, there are problems. HSAs now regulate hospital construction. Dominated by forces ignorant, at best, of mental health needs, and even openly hostile in some locales, government hospital construction is often treated with derision. Private hospitals hire high-power HSA lobbying consultants, establishing a process norm of slick presentations, special pseudosurveys, and excellent PR work. In our experience, public mental health facilities receive very poor treatment. Renewal of physical plant may be difficult or impossible.

The Demand for Public Hospital Beds is likely to Rise Sharply

Just based on demographic factors (Pollack, 1978), one can predict a 25 percent increase in the need for chronic institutional beds during this decade. This estimate is based on the assumption that the illness rate will remain constant and the currently deinstitutionalized will stay out of hospitals. The projected increase is based solely on changes in the age distribution and race distribution of the population.

The actual needs are likely to be far more severe. What has passed for deinstitutionalization is largely a farce. Only one quarter of the community mental health centers on which community care was predicated were ever erected. Moreover, these institutions lack physicians qualified to administer the only treatments thus far demonstrated to have value in treating chronic patients outside the hospital — pharmacologic agents (Pasamanick, 1967). The criticism of the CMHC movement is really as unfair as the criticism of the earlier state hospital movement. Houck (1975) sums up the fate of mental health care institutions well:

> By 1850, the basic patterns of care for the mentally
> ill had already been laid down. There were always more
> sick people than beds to care for them, always more
> expenses than the budget provided, always needs to
> support those who could not support themselves.
> More than a century later, we are still trying to
> solve the same problems with about the same degree
> of success.

Moreover, deinstitutionalization is hardly the exodus from total asylums it was alleged to be. The percentage of Americans living in institutions of all kinds remained constant at 1 percent between 1950 and 1970. While those in state hospitals dropped from 39 percent to 20 percent of the total, those in nursing homes increased from 19 percent to 44 percent of the total (Kohner, 1975, Telhoff, 1979). Why are patients in "nursing homes" instead of hospitals?

The answer to this question creates a new record for cynicism in the care of the mentally ill. The transfer from psychiatric hospitals for chronic mental illness to nursing homes was motivated by a desire to obtain Title XIX money with its 60 percent federal portion, while deluding the public

into thinking this was "deinstitutionalization" and "community care".
Suddenly, total institutions designed and accredited primarily for care of the
elderly and the physically impaired were redefined as "the community".
Movement from a true therapeutic community to a rigid, starched uniform
hospital bed in a nursing home institution was redefined as "deinstitutionalization." Orwell's *1984* contains no worse examples of government dis-
tortion of language to label a phenomenon with its descriptive opposite.
While decades of knowledge and experience about design of humane environments for the chronically mentally ill were ignored, irrelevant codes
governed enormous capital expenditure in building useless institutions.
Doors and windows are designed with correct widths so that patients can
be wheeled out in beds. (Presumably, when fires sweep these new bril-
liantly planned resources, ambulatory psychiatric patients will all jump
on beds and be wheeled around by the staff!) It seems to have dawned
on none of the brilliant code writers that adequate recreation space might
have been preferable, or that different codes might be appropriate for
ambulatory and non-ambulatory patients.

So what happens when the charade stops — when someone reads the
clear intent of the Title XIX regulations and enforces the law — when the
elderly successfully protest that old-age helplessness is tough enough
without the added indignity of being indiscriminantly mixed in a nursing
home with young chronic schizophrenic patients — when an aging population seeks to utilize its nursing homes for what they were designed
for — what then? What happens when the per diem costs under Skilled
Nursing Facility (SNF) rules match those of a well-run chronic hospital?
Will the bureaucrats who engineered and perpetuated the fraud atone for
their guilt by redeveloping correct psychiatric "asylums" — safe places
for the severe chronically impaired? Anyone who really believes that
must be ready for one of those asylums himself! The sorry record of the
past is all too likely to be replayed. From "nursing home" to boarding
home to police lockup to emergency room to acute hospital to boarding
home and over and over until the revolving door spins the patient to the
state hospital.

The trend is as clear as is possible. What has passed for deinstitutionalization is producing a new generation of chronic social-breakdown
syndrome patients, held in a new total institution, the nursing home.
When they are "dumped," as inevitably they will be, the wards of state
hospitals will swell again *unless* we all accept the zone of transition
boarding home of large cities as a preferable next snakepit.

SOME POSSIBLE SOLUTIONS

Can the crisis in in-patient care be averted? Will snakepits inevitably
reappear over the next twenty years? Communities with the will and courage to speak frankly of the level of the danger, the failures of the nos-
trums of the 1960s and 1970s, and the need for prompt action may avert
what otherwise seems to this author inevitable. We recommend the following:

Acute In-patient Services

1. *Psychiatric deployment*. Psychiatrists must be redeployed to
care for the severely ill instead of the worried well. Elsewhere we have
written of neighborhood support systems for "the worried well" (Naper-
stak, Biegel, and Spiro, 1982). Emphasis in training programs, modeling
of socially responsible behavior by teaching institutions, insurance coverage, and special fee structure for treatment of more difficult patients may

encourage needed redeployment.

2. *Standard setting.* Clear standards for psychiatric facilities, equivalent to JCAH standards, must be rigidly enforced. Federal legislation might be considered, which would deprive states of federal health and welfare funds automatically if state hospitals fell below these standards and failed to prove corrective steps were being taken. JCAH standards are at best one key to avoid re-creation of snakepits. Unfortunately, the only "teeth" in current statute is withdrawal of insurance funds, for which the hospitals are largely ineligible. Often the same state department that permits the deterioration is also responsible for determining insurance eligibility. Peer review by a group such as the JCAH is preferable to direct government regulation.

3. *Federal insurance dollars.* Within funding, deterioration of care is inevitable. Direct government funding alone is a poor way to develop hospital care. Government programs tend to be cut back during inflationary cycles. Psychiatric hospitals thus are caught in a squeeze, with inflationary pressures driving costs up even as revenues decrease. This sets in motion a cycle of deteriorating care, which produces the snakepit. Insurance reimbursement can be pegged to rate review processes that reflect the costs required to meet mandated standards of care. It is a shortsighted public policy to exclude psychiatric care from health insurance. Federal laws should *require* that all health insurance include acute hospital coverage in *any* JCAH-accredited acute hospital resource. Discrimination against private psychiatric hospitals merely costs taxpayers money while impairing patient care.

4. *Secondary and tertiary prevention.* The main defense against swelling institutional populations must be early and effective intervention in acute illness (secondary prevention) and programs directed against prevention of chronic institutional-breakdown syndromes (tertiary prevention). Maximal application of therapeutic community principles and efforts to enhance patient autonomy and dignity are the best way to achieve tertiary prevention. (See Spiro, 1980, for review of secondary and tertiary prevention literature.)

5. *PSRO and quality assurance programs.* Often Professional Standard Review Organizations and other quality assurance devices are perceived as a paperwork nuisance by professionals. Indeed, the original purpose of such programs, which was to diminish costs, has not been fulfilled. The programs have proved useful in an entirely different way. Systematized quality assurance programs that produce hard data for legislative groups and for Joint Commission visiting teams are an excellent way to ensure that an asylum does not turn into a snakepit. This is particularly true if the quality assurance programs are mandated and required as part of a federal insurance program that flows only when there is Joint Commission accreditation. Such quality assurance programs can then be enforced through systematic rewards in the form of third-party insurance dollars, which decrease tax levy. In the long run, proper feedback loops that give a prompt "early warning system" will head off problems before they occur. In the past, snakepits were exposed only through effective investigative reporting or the exceptionally brave superintendent who would tell the truth and often lose his head in consequence. Both approaches are too erratic, too undependable, and too late to be effective in maintaining the quality of the in-patient care system.

Subacute and Chronic Care Systems

1. *The regional hospital.* The creation of regional psychiatric hospitals that are fully equipped but are reasonably close to the populations

that they serve may provide sufficient critical mass for programs of excellence. Specialization is a key to effective chronic care. The all-purpose general hospital psychiatry ward will never deal effectively with the subacute and chronic populations. Elsewhere we have suggested that the regional psychiatric facility may serve as a tertiary care program as part of a tri-level system (Spiro, 1969). We believe this to be the best approach to move "on beyond mental health centers" to a true comprehensive system of mental health services. So long as the chronic care system is entirely in the hands of community mental health centers, social myths and community dumping appear to be the dominant themes.

  2. *Psychiatric care in the chronic hospital.* Psychiatric care for patients who require more than 90 days of hospitalization may require intense intervention for periods of up to a year. Borderline states, patients with severe primitive object splitting, and certain schizophrenic patients may be susceptible to successful treatment through this method. The approach must be characterized by a great deal of flexibility. Alternative methods must be tried. Some units should be built around social learning and behavior therapies. Others may be developed around drug-free environments with intensive therapeutic community and even psychoanalytically based interventions. Only in the highly specialized tertiary care hospital are such programs possible. Cost effectiveness of one year of intensive care, even if it can produce a 15 percent remission rate, would be very high in contrast to the expense of having 100 percent of these patients in chronic institutions for an average span of some 35 to 40 years. The myth that every patient must be treated in 14 days and thrown back out in the street must be debunked. The time has come to re-create special "asylums" built on something besides the denial of chronicity. So long as all illnesses are treated as though they were acute, the proper rehabilitation, social learning, psychodynamic, and therapeutic community approaches cannot be developed. The community at large must be educated to understand that such care is more expensive in the short run but potentially far less expensive in the long run than human warehousing and snakepits.

  3. *Alternative systems of care.* Maintenance in the community must no longer be dependent upon creation of inappropriate institutions such as general medical nursing homes. The rehabilitation approach should be based upon fairweather lodges, programs such as Stein's innovative PACT system (Stein, 1978), case management approaches, and other appropriate alterantives to hospitalization. The alternative-to-hospitalization approach has never received a fair trial. The community mental health center was never capable of producing such a system. It was never funded to produce such a system. What passed for deinstitutionalization was "dumping" into total institutions or into boarding homes. In communities like Madison, Wisconsin, the alternative-to-hospitalization system has worked. The author is convinced that similar programs could work effectively in large communities so long as patients were specifically selected for appropriateness. The time has come to cease the "either-or" approach, which provides neither chronic care nor an alternative care system. We must provide both.

  4. *The psychiatric village.* Finally, we believe that patients who need to be institutionalized for more than a year may best be placed in special villages that develop an integral community life of their own. Those who think that this is a return to nineteenth century concepts are quite right. Much of what has been learned in the past is based on very sound principles. The village life, with its farm, its carpentry shops, its special occupations for those who can only remain gainfully occupied in a highly protected environment, is appropriate for a very tiny percentage of severe

chronic schizophrenic patients. It is beyond the scope of this paper to discuss the precise nature of the "sane" asylum for the chronically mentally ill. We believe, however, that the creation of such institutions should become a major agenda for the next decade. The most serious problem in creating such institutions is the precise determination of which patients appropriately belong in them. The number of individuals should be limited. The screening should be extremely stringent. Review of patients on a yearly basis should take place to see which patients can be transferred to more acute treatment environments. Inspection of such villages should be intense and regular to ensure that cruelty, exploitation, and overcrowding, which characterized the forefunners of such institutions, does not recur.

SUMMARY

It would appear that a series of trends render it highly probable that the snakepits of the past will recur in the next two decades. Only a pluralistic system of acute, subacute, and chronic care, composed of a large spectrum of resources, funding mechanisms, and quality assurance mechanisms, can prevent the re-emergence of the snakepit.

REFERENCES

Brill, H. The mental hospital and its patients. *Psych. Annals* 5:9, 1975.

Houck, J.H. The private psychiatric hospital. *Psych. Annals* 5:9, 1975.

Meyer, N.G. Provisional patient movement and administrative data, state and county psychiatric inpatient services. Mental Health Statistical Note 132. Rockville, Maryland: NIMH, 1976.

Naparstek, A., Biegel, D., Spiro, H.R. *Toward, Humane Mental Health Care.* New York: Plenum, 1982 (in press).

Pasamanick, B. et al. *Schizophrenics in the Community.* New York: Appleton-Century-Crofts, 1967.

Sarbin, T. and Mancuso, J. Paradigms and moral judgments: improper conduct is not disease. *J. of Cons. and Clin. Psych.* 39:1, 1972.

Scheff, T.J. *Being Mentally Ill: A Sociological Theory.* New York: Aldine, 1966.

Solomon, H.C. The American Psychiatric Association in relation to American psychiatry. *Am. J. Psych.* 115, July, 1958.

Spiro, H.R. On beyond mental health centers. *Arch. Gen. Psych.* 21, 1969.

Spiro, H.R. Prevention in Psychiatry in Kepken, H., Freedman, A.H., and Scdock, B.S. *Comprehensive Textbook of Psychiatry/III.* Baltimore: Williams and Wilkins, 1980.

Stein, L. *Alternatives to Mental Hospital Treatment.* New York: Plenum, 1978.

Szasz, T.S. *Law, Liberty, and Psychiatry: An Inquiry into the Social Uses of Mental Health Practices.* New York: MacMillan, 1963.

Zilboorg, G. and Henry, G.W. *History of Medical Psychology.* New York: Norton, 1941.

11

Psychiatry in Crisis

David B. Marcotte
Eugenia L. Gullick

SEXUALITY IN THE 1980S

Psychiatry will enter the 1980s beset by identity problems in a number of areas, and a major set of problems in the field of sexuality. Psychiatry seems to be poised in a position between the field's historical underinvolvement in sex education and therapy, and its emerging preoccupation with issues of sexuality — sometimes resulting in a tendency to blur traditional therapist-patient boundaries.

The historical perspective will help to clarify the tenuous position in which psychiatry finds itself. The last several decades have been marked by our culture's growing trend toward openness and interest in sexual functioning. Kinsey (1948, 1953) and Hunt (1974) have demonstrated that we are gradually adopting a more tolerant attitude toward sexual expression. Our "sexual renaissance" (Hunt, 1974) has led to an increase in sex education and open discussion of sexuality. Both Kinsey (1948) and Hunt (1974) have documented the widespread increase in sexual activity and sexual flexibility, focusing on the growing trend toward freedom of choice as an important factor in the development of an individual's sexual practice. The consequence of this emerging openness has been an increasing demand for accurate sex education.

The impact of the "sexual renaissance" on the role of the physician has not been slight. Traditionally, the public has expected physicians to be knowledgeable about sexuality, to provide accurate clinical information, and to assist in the treatment of the sexual dysfunctions. The new openness has led to an increase in sexual questions being asked of the physician. Until recently, most medical schools did not include in their curriculum, course work or training in the area of human sexuality. Therefore, the physician, when asked sexual questions by patients, was left generally unprepared, and frequently used his own behavior as a proscriptive norm for the treatment of others. Many physicians acquired a sense of normality from their own development and behavior. Lief (1970) has indicated that most physicians come from a delayed psychosexual developmental background when compared to the background of those patients they treat. The resulting failure of the physicians to appropriately answer sexual questions has left the public with an uncomfortable choice between requesting assistance from a nonphysician, or denying their questions and problems.

Masters' and Johnson's (1966, 1970) work introduced to the field of sexual functioning a strong element of scientific rigor. Their investigation of the human sexual response and human sexual inadequacy produced a body of scientific knowledge that led to the creation of a short-term, intensive, behavioral treatment of sexual dysfunctions. The impressive success rate of their treatment program represented the first challenge to the psychoanalytical mode of treatment, which has been largely unsuccessful in the amelioration of sexual dysfunctions (Masters and Johnson, 1970). The enthusiasm that followed Masters' and Johnson's discoveries led to a public thirst for more accurate sexual information and more accessible behavior therapy for sexual dysfunctions. At this point, psychiatry had the opportunity to become a strong leader in this trend by disseminating information to patients prophylactically before sexual dysfunctions developed. Instead, psychiatry ignored these demands, and generally persisted in treating sexual dysfunctions in the context of the traditional, long-term psychoanalytical model. This led to a shift in public confidence from psychiatry to more non-physician-led sexual clinics across the country. A plethora of sexual therapy clinics offering short-term, intensive, behavioral interventions proposed by Masters and Johnson (1970), Barbach (1976), and Annon (1974) resulted. This growth pattern represented a mixed blessing for the large number of couples requesting treatment. While it provided a sufficient number of clinics to treat sexual dysfunction, the *quality* of treatment offered was quite variable from clinic to clinic. In some cases the treatment being offered bore no resemblance to that described by Masters and Johnson (1966), Barbach (1976) and Annon (1974), and may have been characterized by such therapeutic interventions as group nudity, sexual activity between patient and therapist, and so on. Ethical concerns about such treatment led to the need for quality control to be applied to sexual dysfunction clinics. Certification of qualified sex therapists has been attempted by a number of organizations. The Society for Sex Therapists and Researchers (SSTR) has made a concerted and quite cautious effort to certify people with expertise in the field. On the other hand, the American Association of Sex Educators, Counselors and Therapists (ASSECT), has cast its net much broader and has certified large numbers of people, including nonprofessionals as well as professional therapists (ASSECT, 1975).

While such strides were being made in the field of sexual therapy, much attention was focused on the need for medical sex education. Dr. Harold Lief (1973), an eminent psychiatrist and psychoanalyst, argued for widespread development of medical sex education. Wood and Natterson (1967, 1969) revealed the widespread ignorance and conservative attitudes that shaped the physician's response to patients with sexual difficulty. Lief (1970) pioneered the development of sex education throughout the United States, so that within a decade most medical schools contained some form of sex education within its curriculum (Holden, 1974). Most of these educational efforts dealt quite successfully with the development of a fund of accurate information and produced attitudinal changes; however, they failed to provide adequate training to assist young physicians in developing management skills and brief therapy technology to deal with sexual dysfunctions clinically. Furthermore, these programs did not extend training to the vast majority of physicians already in practice, and to whom the public was turning for answers to their sexual problems.

At the same time, other cultural developments increased the pressure on the medical profession to provide accurate information regarding sexual functioning. United States public health records indicate that, since 1900, the age of onset of puberty and menses has fallen approximately six years. Consequently, young adults enter into adolescence with an increase in sexual readiness and physical ability to procreate. Furthermore, new developments in medicine have removed old barriers to sexual activity in adolescents and young adults. The availability of legal abortions, the treatment and control of venereal disease, and the availability of contraceptives to minors without parental permission have all served to make sexual activity more accessible to younger and younger teenagers. Additionally, the cultural focus on higher education, which has been apparent since the late 1950s, has led many young people to pursue educational and professional degrees, delaying marriage until a later age. The result of all these changes has been an increase in the number of couples engaging in premarital sexual activities.

Changes in the roles of men and women in our society have further led to alterations in sexual behavior. Increasing attention has been paid to the encouragement of truly pluralistic norms of sexual behavior, which provide for alternative lifestyles and offer a number of sexual options to both married and unmarried couples. The increased incidence of divorce (Reiss, 1980a) since World War II has further contributed to the development of diversity of sexual choices. Recreational sex has become an option, and our culture has begun to view with more tolerance the life-styles of creative singlehood, cohabitation, postdivorce sexual behavior, and sexual activity among the aging in our society. Over the past two decades we have liberalized sexual attitudes to encourage flexibility of sexual expression in all age groups (Christensen, 1970, Reiss, 1980a). In this period of increasing tolerance and acceptance of sexual behavior, the focus has been on the provision of accurate information about sexual functioning and on the freedom of choice of the individual. Christensen (1970) has reported that sexual behavior in the United States closely follows that found in the Scandinavian countries, with a delay factor of between 5 and 10 years. Reiss (1980b) and Clayton (1975) indicate that the 1980s will see the development of much more assertive roles of sexual independence for women, fewer pregnancies, and increasing numbers of divorces, resulting in pressure on psychiatrists to lead in the treatment and prevention of marital and sexual dysfunctions.

A LOOK AT THE FUTURE

Our rapidly changing culture introduces new challenges and implications for the changing role of psychiatry. Our sensitivity to sex-role stereotyping and the changes resulting from this will contribute to more variability in the American family. There should be a higher frequency of dual-career marriages, fewer children, and an increase in the number of couples choosing not to have children. While largely serving to encourage individual expression and freedom of choice, these changes will unquestionably result in stress and will lead to increased demands on mental health professionals to take a leadership role in the development of sexual and relationship treatment.

There will emerge a change in focus in the field of psychiatry. In the 1980s, psychiatry will begin to retreat from its involvement in social problem areas such as poverty and racism as symptoms of societal ills, and will move back toward its medical origin. Even within this change in focus, there is a dichotomy of interests held by members of the profession. Some psychiatrists believe the profession will move in the direction of medicine, and strongly advocate a biological model of psychiatry as the only legitimate role of the psychiatrist; others argue that the psychiatrist has a unique position of leadership in the development of treatment programs aimed at legal and social interventions, as well as the development of effective psychotherapies.

There is a need for extensive improvement in the development of effective sex education and medical sex education programs that go beyond our inadequate attempts in the past. Medical schools across the country must focus considerable effort on the provision of accurate and thorough medical sex education for young physicians to deal with the sexual questions of their patients *and* to provide appropriate referral and/or brief office treatment for some commonly occuring sexual dysfunctions. These educational efforts must emphasize the development of a fund of information, appropriate sexual attitudes, and the acquisition of therapeutic skills for effective intervention.

Further educational efforts must be directed at training mental health professionals, particularly psychiatrists, to treat marital and sexual dysfunctions in short-term behavioral programs. The high incidence of marital and sexual problems (Masters and Johnson, 1970) suggests that there is a need for quantity as well as quality in the development of sexual dysfunction clinics. The failure of psychiatry to meet this challenge will result in an increased public demand and utilization of nonmedical, and frequently unethical and inadequately staffed, clinics. This concern for the development of quality care should lead psychiatry to the pursuit of effective methods of certification of sex therapists. Though SSTR and ASSECT have both been concerned about the provision of careful certification, each group has taken a different position on the criteria required for certification. These issues must be explored more thoroughly and attention must be directed to the development of criteria for eligibility. The process of peer review must be a part of the development of quality control for sex therapy clinics.

In addition to educational efforts, the 1980s should see psychiatry turning its attention to some new therapeutic issues in sexuality. The next ten years will be characterized by continuing research contributing to the recognition of the limits of sex therapy. Work by Kaplan (1974) indicates that most problems of sexual functioning are quite amenable to treatment by short-term behavioral therapy. Historically, short-term sexual treatment has been ideally suited for couples and individuals who have difficulty resulting from misinformation and sexual ignorance, or who suffer from sexual dysfunctions of recent onset. The course of therapy is rendered more lengthy and difficult by those clinical problems that have attitudinally based origins, both in individuals and couples. Furthermore, recent scientific literature (Gullick and Peed, 1980; Money, 1980; Nadelson, 1979) suggests a growing trend toward the examination of other relationship variables contributing to or resulting from difficulties in sexual functioning of the couple. This trend suggests that the mental health professional involved in the treatment of marital and sexual problems will see a steady increase in the frequency of clinical problems that require treatment of sexual dysfunction, as well as intervention into other aspects of the relationship. Investigation of a number of these emerging relationship variables are necessary through controlled studies and logitudinal followup.

The 1980s should bring psychiatry and all of the mental health professions to an adjustment of perspective on the true role of sexual functioning in the development and maintenance of effective relationships. The swaying of the pendulum from denial of sexual functioning as an important factor, to the overemphasis on sexual satisfaction as the sine qua non of relationship success should begin to moderate. Other correlates of "successful" relationships should be examined in the literature and applied to the development of treatment modalities. Research and treatment in this area should investigate the importance of effective communication skills, both sexual and nonsexual, in the development of effective relationships.

We should begin to see intimacy taking on a new and broader definition, and recognize that sexual preference, functioning, and so on, represents only one method of intimacy acquisition.

CRISIS IN DOCTOR-PATIENT SEX

The Hippocratic oath clearly states, "In every house where I come, I will enter only for the good of my patients, keeping myself far from all intentional ill-doing, and all seduction, and especially from the pleasures of love with women and men" (Stedman, 1972). Although this dictum is shared by every professional organization, and violation is rigidly frowned upon, there has been and continues to be a growing difficulty with physicians engaging in sexual activity with their patients (Kardener, Fuller, Mensch, 1973; Marmour, 1972). Never before has a doctor-patient sexual relationship been considered to be a part of the therapeutic contract. With the advent of sex therapy, however, a number of sex therapists have advocated sexual activity with their patients as a necessary component of therapeutic intervention (McCartney, 1966) and argue that it can be beneficial (Shepard, 1971).

Patient-healer or advisor sex behavior is not limited to the medical profession but is found in all other professions (Holroyd, Brodsky, 1977). Difficulty exists in controlling sexual activity between a professional and patient or client because of reluctance on the part of professionals to interfere in a confidential contract, the fear of a law suit, the severity of economic loss to the professional, and the difficulty in substantiating claims of abuse. Particular problems are noted in the control of sexual behavior of psychiatrist and patient because of the reluctance of district branches of psychiatric associations to press for censure of its members (Grunbaum, Nadelson, Macht, 1976). Special sanctions must be developed to protect both patient and professional engaged in sex therapy. Unfortunately, the boundaries that exist to protect both therapist and patient have been blurred by professionals whose own needs are satisfied before those of the patient. Of interest is the fact that the vast majority of reported sexual activity between patient and therapist has been engaged in by male therapists, and the victims largely have been attractive and sexually-appealing females. Contamination of a therapeutic contract by the power needs of the physician are common with the physicians who engages in sexual activity with patients. Advocates for physician-patient sexual activity rationalize that no harm is being done and cite retrospective examples to bolster their claim.

Prospective research, using controlled populations, in which physicians engage in sexual behavior with patients has been proposed (Katz, 1977). The relationship between therapist and patient is confusing when the boundaries are blurred so that the physician loses his/her objectivity and ceases to be an effective sounding board for the patient.

The argument that states that some people engage in sexual contact with their patients and do them no harm can be analogous to the situation surrounding the use of a toxin; when a patient survives the toxic stimulus, they may be all the better equipped to handle subsequent toxic stimuli. Basically the use of one's power and authority over another person (toxin) can hardly help that person choose his own options and reject and respond according to free choice.

The majority of individuals who seek sexual therapy have ongoing relationships and partners. The effective therapist will capitalize on the skill in utilizing the patient and current partners to assist treatment. In cases in which that is not possible, the therapist who utilizes himself or herself as a substitute for the patient effectively establishing other rela-

tionships fosters dependency in the patient, exposes the patient to unrealistic expectations, and also exerts power and control over the patient.

If research is advocated to test the hypothesis that therapist-patient
sexual behavior is beneficial then, in order to alleviate the therapist's
own satisfaction of his needs, several guidelines could be established.
The therapist would not be allowed to select patients for the treatment;
only surrogate partners, not the therapists themselves, could be potential
sexual partners. If such guidelines were established, the issues of patient benefit would, in our opinion, quickly be silenced.

The process of therapy is to enable the patient to become effective
in forming relationships outside the therapeutic relationship, it is not
to be a substitute for effective interpersonal relationships that should
occur outside of the therapeutic relationship.

SUMMARY

What will help in the future? Ideally, nothing can be substituted for
adequate professional judgment and further research in sexual therapy.
The development of valid, reliable instruments that can be used in outcome studies with carefully controlled populations will define the future
direction of the field.

Psychiatry must take a leadership role in certifying qualified sex
therapists. Increasing attention to knowledge of transference and counter-
transference issues in treatment will be necessary for people who enter
into the field of treating sexual dysfunctions. Quality training programs
must be developed with rigorous demands for clear supervision of the
therapist engaging in sexual treatment. Unfortunately, the pressure created by the public demand for treatment has been slow to influence traditional departments of psychiatry throughout the country to develop training programs that provide such experience.

What could hurt psychiatry? As in the past when psychiatry has
failed to take a leadership role in the development or evaluation of treatment techniques, it could fail to lead in the treatment of sexual dysfunctions. If we as a profession neglect the public concern and demand,
other professionals and nonprofessionals will rush to fill that need. We
will therefore have little influence as to which treatment programs are
developed.

In the past the psychiatrist's commitment to develop a multi-disciplinary approach to patient care has sometimes negated our role as experts
in the field of interpersonal relationships and in the medical treatment of
psychological problems. If as a profession we fail to exercise our leadership role in the area of human sexuality, it is possible to see the development of an entire psychosexual health care system that proceeds in directions we believe will be damaging to our patients.

REFERENCES

American Association of Sex Educators, Counselors and Therapists.
    Ethical Standards for Sex Therapists. 1975. Available from AASECT,
    5010 Wisconsin Avenue, N.W., Washington, D.C. 20016.
Annon, J.S. *The Behavioral Treatment of Sexual Problems.* Honolulu,
    Hawaii: Kapioloni Publishers, 1974.
Barbach, L.G. *For Yourself: The Fulfillment of Female Sexuality.* New
    York: Anchor Books, 1975.
Berman, E.M. and Lief, H.I. Marital therapy from a psychiatric perspec-
    tive: An overview. *Amer. J. Psychiat.* 132:583-592, 1974.

Christensen, H.T. and Gregg, C.F. Changing sex norms in America and Scandanavia. *J. Marriage Family* 32:616-627, 1970.

Clayton, R.R. *The Family: Marriage and Social Change.* Lexington, Mass.: Heath and Company, 1975.

Grunbaum, H., Nadelson, C., Macht, L. Sexual activity with the psychiatrist: A district Branch Dilemma. Unpublished Presentation at the American Psychiatric Association Meeting, May, 1976.

Holden, C. Sex therapy: Making it as a science and industry. *Science,* 186:330-334, 1974.

Holroyd, J.C. and Brodsky, A.M. Psychologists' attitudes and practices regarding erotic and nonerotic physical contact with patients. *Amer. Psychologist,* 32:843-49, 1977.

Hunt, M. *Sexual Behavior in the 70s.* Chicago: Playboy Press, 1974.

Kaplan, H.S. *The New Sex Therapy.* New York: Brunner-Mazel, 1974.

Kardener, S.H., Fuller, M., Mensch, I.N. A survey of physician attitudes and practices regarding erotic and nonerotic contact with patients. *Amer. J. Psychiat.* 130:1077-1080, 1973.

Katz, J. Ethical issues in sex therapy and research; Reproductive Research Conference. W. Masters et al (eds). Boston: Little, Brown, 1977.

Kinsey, A.C., Pomeroy, W., Martin, C., Gebhard, P. *Sexual Behavior in the Human Female.* Philadelphia: W. B. Saunders, 1953.

Kinsey, A.C., Pomeroy, W., Martin, C. *Sexual Behavior in the Human Male.* Philadelphia: W.B. Saunders, 1948.

Lief, H.I. Obstacles to the ideal and complete sex education of the medical student and physician. *Contemporary Sexual Behavior: Critical Issues of the 1970s.* J. Zubin and J. Money (eds.), Baltimore: Johns Hopkins Press, 22:441-453.

Lief, H.I. Sex education in medical schools. *J. Med. Educ.* 45:1025-1031, 1970.

Marmour, J. Sexual acting out in psychotherapy. *Amer. J. Psychoanalysis,* 32:3-8, 1972.

Masters, W. and Johnson, V. *Human Sexual Inadequacy.* Boston: Little Brown, 1970.

Masters, W. and Johnson, V. *Human Sexual Response.* Boston: Little Brown, 1966.

McCartney, J. Overt transferences. *J. Sex Research* 32:227-32, 1966.

Money, J. *Love and Love Sickness.* Baltimore: Johns Hopkins Press, 1980.

Nadelson, C.C., Polonsky, D.C., Matthews, M.A. Marriage and midlife: The import of social change. *J. Clin. Psychiat.* 40:293-98, 1979.

Peed, S., Gullick, E., King, L. Some Characteristics of Patients Seeking Sex Therapy. Unpublished manuscript, Medical college of Virginia. Richmond, VA, 1977.

Reiss, I. *Family Systems in America,* 3rd Ed. New York: Holt, Rinehart and Winston, Inc., 1980.

Reiss, I. Sexual customs and gender roles in Sweden and America: An analysis and interpretation. In *The Interweave of Social Roles: Women and Men.* H. Lopato (ed). Greenwhich, Conn: JAI Press, 1980.

Sager, C. *Marriage Contracts and Couple's Therapy.* New York: Brunner-Mazel, 1976.

Shepard, M. *The Love Treatment: Sexual Intimacy Between Patient and Psychotherapist.* New York: Wyden Books, 1971.

Stedman's Medical Dictionary, 22nd Edition. Baltimore: Williams and Wilkins, 1972.

U.S. Bureau of the Census, Current Population Reports. Marital status and living arrangements. Washington, D.C.: U.S. Government Printing Office, March 1976.

Wood, S. and Natterson, J. Sexual attitudes of medical students: Some implications for medical education. *Amer. J. Psychiat.* 124:323-332, 1967.

Woods, S. and Natterson, J. Sexual attitudes of medical students in the psychology of sex: Training in socio-cultural sensitivity. *Amer. J. Psychiat.* 125:1508-1519, 1969.

12

Psychiatry's Changing Role in Medical Education

Sidney Zisook
Richard Devaul

The psychiatrist of the 1980s will have a greatly expanded role in the undergraduate education of physicians. Despite the ever-present struggles for academic recognition, credibility, respect, resources, and, most important, time in the curriculum, departments of psychiatry now have significant teaching responsibilities in the four-year medical curriculum. Both content of psychiatric instruction and teaching techniques, however, are undergoing rapid change. Paradoxically, psychiatry's strength in the medical education curriculum in the 1980s will rely, not on the teaching of *clinical psychiatry*, but rather, on the teaching of humanistic, holistic, person-oriented *medicine*. This chapter discusses the evolving role of psychiatry in medical school education by considering: first, briefly, its history; next, what in particular psychiatry is to teach and why psychiatry as a discipline is best suited to teach it; and, finally, how psychiatry can best achieve these goals for the 1980s within the constraints of the medical education environment.

HISTORY

The history of psychiatry as part of the American medical school curriculum can be divided into roughly four periods: pre-twentieth century, pre-World War II, the post-World War II period through the 1960s, and the decade of the 1970s. Before the twentieth century, infrequent and sporadic attempts to introduce psychiatry into medical education were largely ignored. Benjamin Rush wrote the first textbook on mental diseases in 1812 (Rush, 1812), and Pliny Earle delivered a series of lectures on mental disease at the College of Physicians and Surgeons in 1853, but most schools failed to admit virtually any psychiatry into their curricula (Romano, 1970). The 1871 recommendation of the Association of Medical Superintendents of American Institutions for the Insane that lectures and clinical experience in psychiatry be a part of medical education had little immediate impact.

The authors wish to thank Elizabeth Gammon and Faith Jervey for their research and editorial assistance in the writing of this paper.

The first part of the twentieth century was marked by steady growth in the influence of psychiatry in medical education (Romano, 1970; Webster, 1969). In 1909 the Council of Education of the AMA published a model medical school curriculum that scheduled 30 hours of psychiatry in the senior year (Council on Medical Education, 1909). Three years later, the American Association of Medical Colleges (AAMC) set a standard minimum of 20 hours in psychiatry for its member schools (Franz, 1912). Two surveys of psychiatry in medical education were conducted during the period, the first in 1914 (Graves, 1914) and the second in 1933 (Noble, 1933). A comparison of their results shows that during the intervening years the average number of hours allowed for the teaching of psychiatry increased from 26 to 77 hours and that psychiatry made its first appearance in pre-clinical instruction. The National Committee for Mental Health sponsored four annual conferences between 1933 and 1936 on topics ranging from the formation of an American Board of Psychiatry and Neurology to methods of teaching psychiatry. By 1940, psychiatry was part of the clinical curriculum (average − 72 hours) in all medical schools and part of the pre-clinical curriculum (average − 26 hours) in 88 percent (Ebaugh, 1944).

The part played by psychiatry in the medical care of soldiers during World War II resulted in greater social and political appreciation of psychiatry's potential. Medical education benefited from the new belief in psychiatry, which manifested as increased federal funding for training and research, appropriation of more hours for psychiatry in medical school curricula, and greater numbers of graduates choosing psychiatry as a career. The concurrent mental hygiene movement brought improvement in care in state mental hospitals, introduction of psychiatric services in general hospitals, and the National Mental Health Act of 1946, which created a mechanism for allocation of educational and research funds in psychiatry. With the founding, four years later, of the National Institute of Mental Health (NIMH), the federal government began awarding training grants for the psychiatric education of medical students and the training of psychiatric residents. Ushering in a period of rapid growth in psychiatric education, the NIMH soon suggested programs in behavioral sciences and a variety of other educational programs (Eaton, Daniels, and Pardes, 1977).

The discipline flourished during the next 20 years, most markedly, perhaps, in the 1960s. Objectives and recommendations for the teaching of psychiatry in medical school were formulated at the two Ithaca Conferences in the early 1950s (Whitehorn, 1952), and were later implemented with the support of federal aid (Romano, 1970). In 1956 the Committee on Medical Education of the American Psychiatric Association (APA) recommended 100 hours of psychiatry and behavioral science in the first two years of medical school as a means of sensitizing future physicians to psychosocial factors in health and illness (APA, 1956). Pre-clinical instruction in behavioral science was encouraged further by a 1958 NIMH grant to foster better understanding of the interaction between behavior and health (Group for the Advancement of Psychiatry (GAP), 1962), and in the following year, the first medical school Department of Behavioral Science was formed at the University of Kentucky (Strauss, 1959). Although other such departments have arisen, most behavioral science courses are still co-ordinated and taught chiefly by psychiatrists.

In 1960 the National Board of Medical Examiners introduced psychiatry as a separate subject area in its clinical exam. Along with gains in required and elective curriculum hours, the ensuing decade was characterized by the continued growth in recognition of psychiatry's place in the understanding and treatment of the medically ill as well as the mentally ill (Webster, 1969; GAP, 1962). The report of the Citizens Commission on Graduate Medical Education stressed the importance of behavioral science and clinical psychiatry in holistic primary care (AMA, 1966). This trend was conceptualized by a joint APA and AAMC conference on psychiatry and medical education as a timely counterbalance to the concurrent overspecialization and overreliance on biophysical models of illness in the training of medical students (Robinson and Robinson, 1969). By the end of the 1960s, "relevant" psychiatric education had more to do with teaching psychological medicine than with teaching traditional psychiatry. Four conferences, three sponsored by the National Institute of Child Health and Human Development and one by the National Institute of Health's Division of Physicians' Manpower in 1969 and 1970, led to the formation of the Association for Behavioral Sciences in Medical Education (U.S. DHEW, 1972), whose stated goals are:

1. To promote the application of social and behavioral science knowledge, skills and perspectives in the education and training of physicians, nurses, and other professional persons working in the field of health.
2. To improve the effectiveness, efficiency and quality of health care, the application of social and behavioral science knowledge, skills and perspectives.
3. To encourage the broadening of educational and training practices in the preparation of physicians, nurses and other health professionals.
4. To aid in the continuing education of teachers, clinicians, researchers, and administrators involved in carrying out the above activities.

The early 1970s saw the founding of the Association for Academic Psychiatrists (1971) and the Association of Directors of Medical Student Education in Psychiatry (1975), groups that help provide information exchange, promote educational research, and enhance teaching of psychiatry in medical schools. The rise of behavioral science in this decade is attested to by its becoming the seventh section in Part I of the National Board exam in 1971, and its capturing of federal support for medical student education. The latter was accomplished in the face of declining funds for training in psychiatry and was due to the relevance of behavioral science in the training of primary care physicians (Eaton, Daniels, and Pardes, 1977; Langsley et al., 1977). Such topics as sexuality, thanatology, and interviewing skills found natural places in the multi-disciplinary teaching of basic sciences and psychopathology in the pre-clinical curriculum. The objective of this method, again, was to help students develop a view of the patient as a biopsychosocial being and to establish that view as the basis for a comprehensive approach to diagnosis, prevention, treatment, and management. Summarizing and formalizing the increasing interplay between psychiatry and primary care medicine, the Health Professionals Association Act of 1976 defined psychiatry as an essential supporting discipline and required all trainees to acquire specific psychiatric interviewing and communication skills, knowledge of what they can handle and what they must refer, parameters of psychosomatic and humanistic medicine, and psychological problems secondary to physical illness (Fink, 1977).

The role of psychiatry in medical education has taken a turn, then, since the early 1960s — a time of peak interest in psychiatry per se. While psychiatry's input is now deemed essential for training primary care physicians in the skills, knowledge, and attitudes necessary for holistic care, federal funds for psychiatry have begun to diminish, increments in curriculum time for behavioral science and psychiatry have leveled off, the percentage of students electing psychiatric residencies has declined, and professional as well as public ridicule of psychiatry as a profession has, if anything, escalated (West, 1978).

There is a further twist to this already involved relationship between medicine and psychiatry. At the same time that psychiatry's influence on medicine in the form of behavioral science was seen as a welcome balance to the biomedical model of disease, psychiatry itself was being tempted to, as Leon Eisenberg says, "seek professional respectability" in greater reliance on biological explanations of psychopathologies (Eisenberg, 1979, p.8). Several trends conspired to make biological psychiatry a tempting direction for the discipline to follow. The availability of psychotropic medications for effective treatment of many psychiatric illnesses and the technical and research advances in understanding the biology of functional disorders, coupled with public and professional devaluation of psychiatry as akin to Shamanism and the responding desire to make psychiatry a "hard" discipline by fitting it into the mold of medicine, spurred an avid interest in neurochemical and neurobiological research. The interest is not in line with the course we have been tracing in medicine. "Just as the moment when the rest of medicine is being pressed to expand its horizons to include psychosocial processes," Eisenberg says, "the findings from therapeutic and basic research are steering psychiatry back to the biomedical mainstream...we may trade the one-sidedness of 'brainless' psychiatry of the past for that of a 'mindless' psychiatry of the future" (Eisenberg, 1979, pp8,9).

Some, notably E. Fuller Torrey (1978), have hypothesized that psychiatry's continued movement along its current course could lead to its dissolution: the concerns that are presently within its province becoming, at one extreme, the domain of neurology, and at the other, of education. Those with diseases of the brain would become patients of the neurologist and those without would be educated or directed in self-education by nonphysicians. The coming decade will challenge psychiatry to resolve this question of its own identity and destiny, and interact effectively with other disciplines in the teaching and practice of medicine. One possible definition of psychiatry's new role is suggested in the very statement of its hypothesized dissolution. Psychiatry does indeed have a biological and an educational component. This has been the source of its strength. The traditional psychotherapeutic model is the paradigm of enlightened doctor-patient relationships, and psychiatry need neither apologize for their orientation nor abandon it. Neurobiology, for its part, will continue to turn out new information and, as L. Jolyon West sees it, the psychiatrist will be called upon to serve as "creative integrator," integrating the new information from biology with empirical behavioral science and applying the results in treatment of those experiencing physical, mental, or emotional distress (West, 1978).

It can be seen that this resolution of psychiatry's internal problem is consonant with the role it is to assume in external relationships also. It will be a difficult role in which fewer psychiatrists with less financial support will be called upon to teach more students in an often hostile arena. Before we look at ways to approach this difficult role, however, three more basic questions must be answered. We have established that psychiatry is taught in medical schools. We must consider why it should be taught and by psychiatrists, what, in fact, is or ought to be taught, and how it can best be taught. We can then return to the issue of whether psychiatry can fulfill such a role within the constraints of the medical educational environment of the 1980s.

WHY TEACH PSYCHIATRY

The preceding brief history traced the initial recognition of psychiatry as a necessary part of medical training and the emergent change in the nature of its contribution. The new emphasis on psychosocial medicine is responsible for psychiatry's changing role, and two newly acknowledged medical needs are, in turn, responsible for the emphasis on psychosocial medicine. The first is the renewed awareness of the need for primary care physicians who will consider the whole patient, indeed, the whole family and its evolving medical history, and provide the continuity of longitudinal care. We have commented on this at some length already but have not explained the situation that forced the re-attention to humanistic care. The results of the technological revolution — scientific discoveries, technical advances, early specialization, sub- and tertiary specialization, and the emergence of group practice with its businesslike trappings — created an image of the medical profession as impersonal, uncaring, and motivated by profit. Individuals and public groups indicted the profession for overlooking "the human side" and for treating "diseased organs" rather than people with illness problems. The 1967 Citizens' Commission on Graduate Medical Education Report's formal naming of the shortage of primary care physicians as the leading problem confronting the medical system helped divert funds, energy, attention, and, most important, new physicians into primary care fields, and identified psychiatry as a major support specialty in the endeavor (AMA, 1966).

By 1974, one-fourth of all U.S. physicians were in primary care fields (Goldberg et al., 1976), which is not to say that they possessed the necessary knowledge and skills to treat the patient-as-a-whole-person optimally. Very little illness, especially in that encountered by the primary care physician, is simple uncomplicated body pathology or injury. Most illness, and certainly all serious illness, is complicated by emotional reaction; in some illness, no organic etiology can be found to account for the complaint; and in all complaints, ethnicity, social setting, and personality affect the degree of distress experienced by the patient (Engel, 1977). Patient noncompliance and dissatisfaction with the doctor-patient interaction can often be explained by sociocultural facts and unrealistic patient expectations (Kleinman, Eisenberg, and Good 1978). These various contributors to illness often go largely unrecognized or ignored. Most patients with emotional problems are initially treated in the outpatient primary care sector of the health system (Goldberg et al., 1976; Regier, Goldberg, and Taube, 1978), where many physicians feel unprepared to handle such problems (Callen and Davis, 1978; Fisher, 1978). More than 50 percent of the prescriptions for psychotropic agents are filled by non-psychiatric physicians, and approximately 12 percent of all physician visits result in prescriptions for sedatives or anti-anxiety agents (Balter, 1973), attesting, at least partially, to physicians' inability to deal with psychosocial problems more directly. Knowledge in behavioral science and training in the skills necessary for the practice of "human" medicine are essential tools for the primary care physician and mandate the teaching of psychosocial medicine in the clinical and basic science curricula of medical schools.

The second medical need that has pressed for the teaching of psychosocial medicine in medical schools is the ascendency of chronic illness as a major medical problem. The place of acute disorders as the greatest killers of mankind has been assumed by heart disease, strokes, and cancer. Chronic illness and technology's means for prolonging the life of the chronically ill present ethical dilemmas heretofore unknown in medical practice — decisions regarding termination of mechanical support systems ("pulling the plug," as it has flippantly been called), choosing one from among many to receive an organ transplant, assessing the cost — benefit ratio of massive chemotherapy, and so on. Making such judgments calls for expansion of the diseased-organ perspective to include psychological, familial, sociological, anthropological, and, certainly, ethical points of view.

The less dramatic, day-to-day management of chronic illness also demands psychosocial sophistication. Here psychological, sociological, and cultural components of illness become at least as important as biological input, often creating marked disparity between reported discomfort on one hand, and structural or functional impairment on the other (Eisenberg, 1979). In treatment of the chronically ill or disabled, the relationship between physician and patient becomes paramount. The physician's role changes from curer of disease to educator and medical psychotherapist, teaching patients to take responsibility for their illness and its management (Parsons, 1951; Szasz and Hollender, 1956). Learning to maximize the potential therapeutic power of the doctor-patient relationship, particularly in less responsive chronic illness, demands a re-orientation on the physician's part that is best begun very early in medical training.

While the psychosocial approach we have been discussing *need* not be presented by psychiatry, psychiatrists as physicians with special understanding of intrapsychic and interpersonal motivation are best suited for the teaching role. The psychiatrists' advantage over the behavioral scientists consists in the formers' knowledge of medicine and experience in hospital work, their being more obvious role models for future physicians, and their roots in neurobiology and clinical medicine. They have an advantage over nonpsychiatrist physicians, also, inasmuch as their specialty training has emphasized the many aspects of the whole patient that psychosocial medicine must address. Clinical interviewing and the doctor-patient relationship, moreover, are cornerstones of psychiatric intervention. The mutual participation model of doctor-patient interaction, the most fitting model for managing chronic illness, has been likened to the model of psychotherapy (Parsons, 1951; Szasz and Hollender, 1956). The integration of biological, psychological, and social perspectives, and the educational rather than healing function that epitomize the psychiatrist's role are precisely the attributes needed for the teaching (and practicing) of the art and science of medicine in the coming decades.

WHAT TO TEACH

The task of translating these rather abstract teaching goals into actual course content is complicated by several problems. The information bases of the behavioral sciences and clinical psychiatry have expanded rapidly over the past two decades and continue to do so, making adequate instruction in all the material impossible within the limits set by the curriculum. This problem is exacerbated by the absence of consensus on what subject areas and topics can be selected, from the unwieldy information bases, as most indispensible and significant. Discussion of behavioral science and psychiatry course content (APA, 1956; Lansley et al., 1977; Bandler, 1969; Brownstein et al., 1977; Dacey and Wintrob, 1973; Lazerson, 1976; Orleans and Houpt, 1978; Steele, 1978; Wexler, 1976) are characterized by agreement only that psychosocial medicine be taught. In reviewing the teaching of only behavioral science in medical schools, Fletcher found 1,294 different course titles and designations in 112 catalogues, an average of 11.6 entries per school (Fletcher, 1974). The Four Conferences on Behavioral Sciences in Medical Education suggested in 1971 that, at a minimum, the skills and principles represented by psychology, sociology, cultural anthropology, and social psychology be part of medical education. The report specified further "a few of the behavioral science concepts and techniques that physicians particularly *need to know* in order to provide true health care," including the presence or absence of the father in the family, principles of human and animal behavior, and such theories of social organization as value orientation, equilibrium, competition, and small and large organization processes (U.S. DHEW 1972; pp. 103-143). The range and choice even here seems wide and somewhat random.

The National Board of Medical Examiners sets standards for evaluation of individual programs and offers general curriculum guidelines by listing topics that are covered by the behavioral science and psychiatry exams (National Board of Medical Examiners, 1979). The list (Table 1) is so inclusive as to be virtually meaningless to curriculum officers who must design coursework for approximately 100 pre-clinical hours and four- to eight-week clinics.

Bowen and Barton's review of literature on the goals of medical student psychiatry education reported, amid varied departmental objectives, agreement that training should include "knowledge of clinical psychopathology, interactions of emotional factors with physiologic functions in health and illness, skills in the doctor-patient relationship and factual knowledge from basic anthropology, biological/psychological and sociological aspects of the behavioral sciences" (Bowden and Barton, 1975). They also found unanimity in the belief, expressed differently by different sources, that there be emphasis on the art of medicine and an appreciation for the human side of biology.

With consensus only on great and undefined areas of knowledge, educators in psychiatry are left to select for themselves what is relevant and digestible in the time frame within which they must work. Resources, faculty skills, student body, and social milieu of the particular institution must bear upon curriculum choices also. Finally, as Reiser points out, the principles psychiatrists choose to teach must "provide a conceptual, schematic matrix into and onto which they can superimpose, fit and integrate all of the new information that is sure to emerge in the years ahead as the interaction explosion continues" (Reiser, 1973).

If, in making medical curriculum decisions, one considers the theoretical goals we have been espousing throughout, while using the institutional concern just mentioned for a foothold in reality, certain fundamentals will, we think, be recognized as basic and indispensible to the practice of psychosocial medicine. These fundamentals are of three orders: knowledge, skills, and attitudes. Of the formidable *knowledge* base that underlies psychiatry and behavioral science, future primary care physicians should certainly know the rudiments of psychopathology, the contents and relevance of the mental status exam, the indications for and limitations of psychotropic agents, the types of problems and people they can deal with comfortably, when to consult with other specialists, and when to refer. They should develop an ethical framework on which to base decisions. Additionally, students should learn about the interaction of psychological, social, and cultural factors with health and illness behaviors. They should understand the different models of doctor-patient relationship and the importance of longitudinal care.

The *skills* are primarily those needed for interacting with a variety of patients while retaining sensitivity in professional encounters. In practical terms, these skills are demonstrated most noticeably in the interview. While it is not necessary for all future physicians to be accomplished psychotherapists, it is necessary for them to incorporate the interviewing, interpersonal relating, and teaching principles of psychotherapeutic management into clinical interactions with patients. In this way psychiatry may be considered the paradigmatic specialty for all of medicine (Eisenberg, 1979).

Attitudes make up perhaps the most important category of the three. Openmindedness, flexibility, inquisitiveness, nonjudgmental caring, and self-reflection are imperative. They are manifestations of the deep sense of humanity, compassion, and personal relationship that is requisite of good physicians. The orders or categories of instruction overlap, of course. Where it is needful to impart *knowledge* — specific facts — the greatest value may be a change in *attitude* or *skills*, effected by the information. For example, sociocultural dimensions of health care are particularly pertinent in primary care today. While lectures may focus on the problems and needs of a particular local population, these group-specific facts are secondary in significance to the students' growing sensitivity to the dynamic impact of cultural influences on any culture's use of medical care. Similarly, encyclopedic knowledge or even exemplary attitudes cannot replace specific problems-solving *skills* when faced with difficult clinical situations.

HOW TO TEACH BEHAVIORAL SCIENCES AND PSYCHIATRY

Instruction in behavioral science, even more than that in clinical psychiatry, has been criticized by students as dull, irrelevant, incoherent, esoteric, and "soft". Its teachers have been censured for taking the self-righteous position of belonging to the only discipline concerned with human values. Students who find some, or even most, of the material interesting, frequently have difficulty translating the wealth of information into specific skills. Others may be confused about how the subject matter will help them survive medical school or become competent physicians. Often the concepts basic to development and behavior are viewed as either too complicated or just plain common sense, and study time for the "real sciences" is allowed to pre-empt attendance at behavioral science lectures. Because behavioral science concepts and interviewing skills are taught, for the most part, by departments of psychiatry, students tend to isolate the knowledge as "psychiatry" and fail to carry the information and attitudes into other services. Finally, with a last nod to the dead horse — inadequate curriculum hours — we move on to acknowledge that the value of behavioral science is subtly undermined by the attitudes of administrators and faculty. These are the problems to which any plan for the teaching of psychiatry and behavioral science must speak.

The misunderstandings and poor attitudes (of both students and teaching staff) should be one of the first problems attacked. If psychiatry departments are to exemplify what they teach, they cannot hold their discipline and its tenets as alone sacrosanct. They must develop positive relationships with other departments and with students. The deteriorating alliance between teacher and student can be revitalized by the department's respect and acceptance for medical student concerns and its consideration of student expectation. Clear-cut objectives should be established and understood. Small groups of students should meet with an instructor for discussions and questions; the latter answered openly and honestly. Socializing out of class should be encouraged as an aid to a "holistic" understanding on the part of the student as more than a classroom learning entity.

Interdepartmental relationships and co-operative teaching must be improved and expanded. Interdisciplinary instruction works both ways. Behavioral science considerations aid comprehension of basically clinical patient problems. For example, a medical/psychosocial discussion of cariovascular disease, jointly presented by behavioral science, psychiatry, cardiology, and possibly community medicine, could incorporate topics relevant to each of those disciplines. Issues in the cardiovascular case example that relate to behavioral science and psychiatry might include life-styles and personality factors, including Type A and B personalities; life cycle considerations, including childhood nutrition, constitutional and genetic factors, illness onset, chronic illness, invalidism and rehabilitation, and death and grief; preventive programs; behavior modification; ethical decisions in use of life supports; sexual concomitants of illness; anxiety, denial, and depression; compliance; epidemiology and experimental animal studies; the need for and limitations of hospitalization; coping; illness behavior and the sick role; the effects of illness on the family; and the doctor-patient relationship (Kimball, 1975).

Likewise, help in behavioral science instruction can come from other departments. The pediatrician, family practitioner, and gerontologist can aid in the teaching of growth and development; internists can demonstrate diagnostic interviewing techniques; obstetricians and urologists can discuss human sexuality. Material relating not only to illness but to normal development and behavior should be integrated with clinical problems and disease entities whenever possible.

An extremely beneficial heuristic undertaking, and one that cuts across many clinical disciplines, is a program of well-supervised student contact with a patient or family over four years time. The following of a family over this period, with necessary consultations, referrals, and followups, resembles the primary care physician's function as closely as any experience medical school can offer, and is the best teacher of the doctor-patient relationship.

Interviewing is doubtless one of the most important of the physician's skills. If it is to amount to more than mere history-taking, interviewing should be introduced early, taught conjointly with medical and surgical clinical faculty, and reinforced continually during the four years. Faculty workshops on "teaching and interviewing skills" may advance the goal of interdepartmental co-operation.

On the clinical training level, multiple settings for psychiatry clerkships are essential. While on psychiatry, students should, ideally, rotate through ambulatory centers, the emergency room, child and community mental health services, and consultation-liaison services. Some opportunity to work with those patient groups that the primary care physician will see most frequently — those, for example, on adolescent units, alcohol or drug treatment units, behavioral medicine units, and geriatric units — should be made available. While on nonpsychiatry rotations, students should continue to interface with the liaison service whenever consult is obtained for their assigned patients.

In fact, the teaching program ideally centers around the consultation-liaison program. Consultation-liaison psychiatry, as the clinical component of psychosomatic medicine, embodies the holistic approach to medicine and shares the teaching orientation of medical education. The competent liaison psychiatrist uses the skills and knowledge all physicians should master: interviewing and diagnostic skills and a knowledge of psychosocial contributors to illness, the importance of the physician-patient relationship, and the influence of personality factors on management. Consultation-liaison psychiatry as it interacts with all other services can be viewed as a model for the psychosocial aspect of the art of medicine, which interacts with biological science and technology to produce medical care. As such, liaison psychiatry is an invaluable aid in the training of humanistic primary care physicians (Lipowski, 1967; 1977).

Finally, the lack of standardized principles of how and what to teach in psychiatry in medical school calls, at once, for innovation and strict evaluation. Objectives must be continually re-evaluated. When objectives are agreed upon, the strategies for achieving them must be defined, evaluated, and themselves revised whenever they seem to be failing the goals. Comparisons between the achievements of individual programs might offer one means of evaluation. The innovations and experimentation that the field allows and that the changing practice of medicine demands from psychiatry will help vitalize medical education in the coming decades.

TABLE I

1. Behavioral Biology	3. Interpersonal and Group Behavior
a. biochemical correlates of behavior	a. adaptation
b. biostatistics	b. attitudes and beliefs
c. comparative behavior	c. child rearing practices
d. genetics of behavior	d. communication (both verbal and nonverbal)
e. pharmacologic correlates of behavior	e. interaction
f. physiologic correlates of behavior	f. leadership
g. psychophysiology	g. physician-patient relationships
	h. prejudice
2. Individual Behavior	i. roles
a. emotions	4. Culture and Society
b growth and development	
c. learning processes	a. community
d. life cycle	b. ethics and law
e. motivation	c. ethnomedicine
f. perception, cognition, and memory	d. family
g. personality	e. health care systems
h. psychodynamics	f. human ecology
i. psychological assessment	g. norms and values
j. psychopathology	h. social institutions and organizations
k. sexual behavior	i. social problems
	j. stratification

CONCLUSION

This discussion of psychiatry's history as part of the medical education curriculum in the United States, what is taught, why, and how, has uncovered many of the crises psychiatry faces in the 1980s. Psychiatry is being asked to take an ever greater role in teaching medical students to practice better medicine. The assignment is being accepted, but, beyond broad theoretical agreement, there is no consensus on which specific facts, skills, and attitudes from the extensive and growing information base relate most closely to the practice of good medicine. Many psychiatrists are uncomfortable in the basic science milieu and out of touch with much of the material generated by the information explosions in behavioral science and neurobiology. Concomitantly, many would like to feel more secure in their knowledge of the "medical" problems encountered by nonpsychiatrist colleagues (Strain, 1977). Whereas more time for reading and study would allow academic psychiatrists to narrow the gap between psychiatry and medicine, they are already taxed by being the only clinicians responsible for teaching their own basic science. The presence of more academic psychiatrists on medical school faculties would alleviate time and work pressures, but fewer are on the horizon. And academic psychiatrists, like other academicians, face administrative, clinical, research, and publishing obligations.

The internal pulling of traditional psychiatry toward a neurobiological model at one end and a purely psychosociocultural one at the other further complicates the execution of its academic task. This struggle suggests the need for psychiatry to resolve its own identity diffusion before it can optimally educate others. Psychiatry can find its rightful medical role without eschewing its psychosomatic underpinnings by continuing to care for chronically and severely disabled individuals, devoting more time to liaison work on medicine and surgery units, delivering care in secondary and tertiary treatment centers, and, most important, supplying teachers and role models for the incorporation of sound psychiatric principles into medical care.

Resolution of the conflict between greater need for instruction in psychosocial medicine and fewer resources in time, teachers, and money to provide it lies in the integration of psychiatry and behavioral science instruction with all other medical instruction. Despite the problems outlined above, psychiatry remains the discipline best suited to teach the kind of psychosocial approach to diagnosis and longitudinal management that medical practice presently demands, but its contribution cannot be isolated from the remainder of the student's education. As practitioners of a specialty closely related to both medicine and behavioral science, yet on the periphery of each, psychiatrists are well situated for directing the interaction of the two. The psychiatrist's role will be to co-ordinate a team approach to the teaching of person-oriented medicine by enlisting co-operation from many departments of instruction. Together, these faculty members can provide comprehensive learning experiences that encompass all medical problems and all aspects of medical care. Psychiatrists are not the only humanists on medical school faculties, the only educators sensitive to psychosocial issues of health care, or the only clinicians who know how to interview patients. As directors of multidisciplinary endeavors, psychiatrists can maximize the time they have for their own learning and growth while overseeing the introduction of the principles of psychiatry into the mainstream of medical education. This must be the goal and the course for the 1980s.

REFERENCES

American Medical Association, Citizens' Commission on Graduate Medical Education Report. Chicago: American Medical Association, 1966.

American Psychiatric Association, Committee on Medical Education. An outline for a curriculum for teaching psychiatry in medical school. *J. Med. Ed.* 31: 115-122, 1956.

Balter, M.B. An analysis of psychotherapeutic drug consumption in the United States. *Anglo-American Conference on Drug Abuse* 1: 58-65, 1973.

Bandler, B. Summary report of the preparatory commission on content. In *Teaching Psychiatry in Medical School*, R. and M. Robinson, (eds). Washington, D.C.: American Psychiatric Association, 1969, pp. 306-309.

Bowden, C. and Barton D. Goals of medical student psychiatric education. *J. Med. Ed.* 50: 257-263, 1975.

Brownstein, E.J., Singer, P., Dornbush, R., Lilienfeld, D.M., Shaker, R., and Freedman, A.M. A behavioral science curriculum for medical students: One model. *J. Psychiatric Ed.* 1: 52-62, 1977.

Callen, K. and Davis, D. The general practitioner: How much psychiatric education? *Psychosomatics* 19:409-413, 1978.

Citizens' Commission on Graduate Medical Education Report. Chicago: American Medical Association, 1966.

Council on Medical Education. A model medical curriculum: A report of a committee of one hundred leading educators of the United States and Canada assisted by many others acting in an auxiliary capacity. *A.M.A. Bull.* 5, 1909.

Dacey, M.L. and Wintrob, R.M. Human behavior: The teaching of social and behavioral sciences in medical schools. *Soc. Sci. & Med.* 7:943-957, 1973.

Eaton, J.S. Jr., Daniels, R.S., and Pardes, H. Psychiatric education: State of the art, 1976. *Am. J. Psychiat.* 134:2-6, 1977.

Eaton, J.S., Jr. and Goldstein, L.S. Psychiatry in crisis. *Am. J. Psychiat.* 134:642-645, 1977.

Ebaugh, F.G. The history of psychiatric education in the United States from 1844-1944. *Am. J. Psychiat.* 100:151-161, 1944.

Eisenberg, L. Interfaces between medicine and psychiatry. *Comp. Psychiatry* 20:1-14, 1979.

Engel, G.L. The need for a new medical model: A challenge for bio-medicine. *Science* 196:129-136, 1977.

Fink, P.J. The relationship of psychiatry to primary care. *Am. J. Psychiat.* 134:126-129, 1977.

Fisher, J.V. What the family physician expects from the psychiatrist. *Psychosomatics* 19:523-527, 1978.

Fletcher, C.R. Study of behavioral science teaching in schools of medicine. *J. Med. Ed.* 49:188-189, 1974.

Franz, S.I. The present status of psychology in medical education and practice. *JAMA* 58:909-911, 1912.

Goldberg, R.L., Haas, M.R., Eaton, J.S. Jr., and Grubbs, J.H. Psychiatry and the primary care physician. *JAMA* 236:944-945, 1976.

Graves, W.W. Some factors tending toward adequate instruction in nervous and mental diseases. *JAMA* 63:1707-1713, 1914.

Group for the Advancement of Psychiatry. Report No. 54, The Pre-clinical Teaching of Psychiatry. New York, 1962.

Kimball, C.P. The clinical case method in teaching comprehensive approaches to illness behavior. *Psychosomat. Med.* 37:454-467, 1975.

Kleinman, A., Eisenberg, L., and Good, B. Culture, illness and care: Clinical lessons from anthropologic and cross-cultural research. *Ann. of Intern. Med.* 88:251-258, 1978.

Langsley, D., Freedman, A.L., Haas, M., and Grubbs, J.H. Medical student education in psychiatry. *Am. J. Psychiat.* 134:15-20, 1977.

Lazerson, A.M. The psychiatrist in primary medical care training: A solution to the mind-body dichotomy? *Am. J. Psychiat.* 133:964-966, 1976.

Lipowski, Z.J. Psychosomatic medicine in the seventies: An overview. *Am. J. Psychiat.* 134:233-244, 1977.

Lipowski, Z.J. Review of consultation psychiatry and psychosomatic medicine. *Psychosomat. Med.* 29:153-171, 1967.

National Board of Medical Examiners. Bulletin of Information and Description of Examination. Philadelphia, 1979, pp. 22-23.

Noble, R.A. Psychiatry in medical education. New York: National Committee for Mental Hygiene, 1933.

Orleans, C.S. and Houpt, J.L. Undergraduate psychiatry education 1971-1976: Trends and findings. *J. Psychiatr. Ed.* 2:146-169, 1978.

Parsons, T.   Illness and the role of the physician: A sociological per-
spective.   *Am. J. Orthopsychiatry* 21:452-460, 1951.
Regier, D.A., Goldberg, I.D., and Taube, C.A.   The de facto U.S.
mental health services system.   *Arch. Gen. Psychiatry* 35:685-
693, 1978.
Reiser, M.F.   Psychiatry in the undergraduate medical curriculum.
Am. J. Psychiat. 130:565-567, 1973.
Robinson, R. and Robinson, M. (eds.).   *Teaching Psychiatry in
Medical School.   The Working Papers of the Conference on Psy-
chiatry and Medical Education, 1967.*   Washington, D.C.:
American Psychiatric Association, 1969.
Romano, J.   The teaching of psychiatry to medical students: Past,
present and future.   *Am. J. Psychiat.* 126:99-110, 1970.
Rush, B.   *Medical Inquiries and Observations Upon the Diseases of
the Mind.*   Philadelphia: Kimber and Richardson, 1912.
Steele, T.E.   Teaching behavioral sciences to medical students: Edu-
cation or training?   *Arch. Gen. Psychiatry* 35:27-34, 1978.
Strain, J.J.   The medical setting: Is it beyond the psychiatrist?
Am. J. Psychiat. 134:253-256, 1977.
Strauss, R.   A department of behavioral science.   *J. Med. Ed.* 34:662-
666, 1959.
Szasz, T.S. and Hollender, M.H.   A contribution to the philosophy of
medicine: The basic models of the doctor-patient relationship.
Arch. Intern. Med. 97:585-592, 1956.
Torrey, E.F.   The Future of Psychiatry is bleak at best.   In
Controversies in Psychiatry.   J.P. Brady and H.K.H. Brodie (eds.).
Philadelphia: W.B. Saunders & Co., 1978, pp. 3-12.
U.S. Department of Health, Education and Welfare.   Behavioral Sciences
and Medical Education: A Report of Four Conferences.   National
Institute of Child Health and Human Development.   Washington,
D.C.: U.S. DHEW Publication No. (NIH) 72-41, 103-143, 1972.
Webster, T.G.   Psychiatry and behavioral science curriculum hours in
the United States schools of medicine and osteopathy.   In *Teaching
Psychiatry in Medical Schools: Working Papers of the Conference on
Psychiatry and Medical Education, 1967.*   Washington, D.C.:
American Psychiatric Association, 1969, pp. 259-288.
West, L.J.   The future of psychiatry is bright.   In *Controversies in
Psychiatry.*   J.P. Brady and H.K.H. Brodie (eds.).   Philadelphia:
W.B. Saunders & Co., 1978, pp. 28-38.
Wexler, M.   The behavioral sciences in medical education: A view from
psychology.   *Amer. Psychologist* April, 1976, pp. 275-283.
Whitehorn, J.G. (ed.).   *Psychiatry and Medical Education.*   Report
of the 1951 Conference on Psychiatric Education held at Cornell
University, Ithaca, New York, 1951.   Washington, D.C.: American
Psychiatric Association, 1952.

13

Aging, The Aged, and Psychiatry: Cinderella Revisited

Alvin J. Levenson
Judy Baggett Thrasher

Bulacratta rolled over sluggishly as a loud crash from the kitchen roused her from a deep sleep. The bed groaned beneath her grotesque weight.

"Can't you be quiet out there? I'm trying to get some sleep so I'll look beautiful for Prince Charming tonight," she said as her fat features forced themselves into a yawn.

"My God, Bula. Why can't you lose weight? Prince Charming will never look at you when your're so fat. Sleep isn't going to help." At one time Jaypea has been a beautiful woman, but years of hard living had aged her quickly and lined her face. Even the heavy makeup she wore couldn't conceal the harshness, and her taunt cold eyes never showed an indication of compassion. As usual she smoothly exited the room before Bula could even think of a retort. Jaypea always had the last word.

The tenseness in the room was broken as the evening paper hit the slightly ajar screen door, slamming it with a bang. Hippocrata was glad of an excuse to leave her bickering sisters as she ran outside and leaned over the white picket fence to yell at the paper boy. The white frame house behind her looked much like every other house on the block. The neighborhood emanated a comfortable air, not rich but not poor. Most of the residents planned to work hard and someday reap the rewards of a comfortable retirement provided by the government and their employer. They would have been shocked to learn the secrets of 65 Overhill Drive.

"Now, now everybody. Let's try to get along," soothed Dulce.

Actually she didn't care if they argued or not, but she didn't want the neighbors to hear. Though she liked to give the appearance of family harmony, every so often her sweet outward demeanor was shattered by a terrifying anger. Most

The author wishes to thank Dianna M. Porter, M.A. (Gerontology) for her assistance in data collection and Mrs. Janet S. King for her preparation of the manuscript.

of the time, however, she was able to coat her anger with a
covering of sweet understanding. Her stepsister felt the
brunt of her pent-up hostilities most often, and even then
Dulce immediately felt guilty for exploding at the old woman.

Evening approached and the four sisters began to dress
for the Ball. Each had a sparkling gown and had spent
hours having their hair curled. All of them hoped to catch
the eye of the Prince. Each had her own reasons for want-
ing him.

"Cinderella! Isn't supper ready yet? I'm hungry,"
yelled Bula as she finally rolled out of bed. "What have
you been doing all this time?"

Cinderella rose wearily from scrubbing the floor and
slowly shuffled to the stove. When she first moved to 65
Overhill, she fought the sisters bitterly. The four women
were too much for her; perhaps if there had only been one
or even two she could have stood up to them. But now,
she had no strength left to do so. She complied with whatever they ordered for, little by little, her resistance had
been chipped away. She felt old. Old and tired. She was
a painfully thin woman with stringy gray hair that was seldom brushed. Rheumatism made it difficult to lift her arms
very high, and Hippocrata told her it was useless to go to
the doctor for the pain. Her clothing was not only old and
tattered, but dirty as well.

"It's almost on the table, stepsister," she called. She
fingered her rags and sighed. Bula and Jaypea kept a
close watch on any money they gave her to run the house,
and no matter how she begged for more they told her she
must make do with what she had.

"I guess they're right," she thought. "What does an
old woman like me need new clothes for anyway? I can't
get a job. Jaypea said nobody would hire me. I never
get to go anywhere, not even to the Ball, since I came
to 65 Overhill."

Bula's shriek brought her thoughts to an abrupt end.
"Is this all we have to eat? What do you do with all the
money?"

"I'm sorry. Prices have gone up since you made that
budget for me. It won't work anymore."

The others sat down at the table just in time to hear the
end of the dispute.

"You're lucky we let you stay here at all and give you
money," said Hippocrata. She was a thin wirey woman with
an air of uncertainty, perhaps resultant of her poor education.
Cinderella, for some reason, made her uncomfortable. "We
could put you away in a home to die, isn't that right?"

Cinderella trembled inside. These four women were her
only link with life, her only way to stay alive. She had to
please them.

"Oh, quit bothering her. She's too old to worry about,"
said Dulce.

"She is already senile," said Hippocrata. They spoke in
front of her as though she couldn't hear them. "I don't even
think modern medicine can help her."

Cinderella ran sobbing from the room.

"I'll give her a couple of those pills Hippocrata got for her," said Dulce sweetly. "They calm her."

Cinderella held the pill under her tongue until Dulce left the room. For months, hiding the pill had been her only form of rebellion. No one had discovered it yet. The pills made her groggy and disoriented; she hated them. She didn't dare let the stepsisters know she wasn't swallowing them though.

She looked at herself in the mirror until she heard the door slam as the sisters left. I look like an old crazy woman, she thought. Is this all that is left to my life?

She crept into the kitchen and surveyed the mess with dismay. But just as she began to gather the dirty dishes, a soft knock sounded on the front door.

"Hello, is anyone home?"

Cinderella hesitated, then opened the door a crack to see a woman her own age. But this woman created a marked contrast to Cinderella. She was neat and clean, her hair tidily caught back in an attractive bun. She held her head high, and entered the kitchen with an air of determination.

"I heard yelling from the street. It reminded me of something in my past, so I had to see for myself if you were okay."

"Okay as I'll ever be."

"What kind of attitude is that?" the woman asked angrily.

"I'm tired. I'm scared. I just can't fight anymore."

"That's stupid. You're giving up, just like they want you to. Exactly as I did for a long time."

"But they'll kick me out. What will happen then? What if they put me in a home?" Tears streamed down her face at the thought.

"I make it alone and I'm happier. You need to do something to be happier too. Remember how things were for grandparents? They had an important part in the family. But times have changed, society is turning from the older person. Nobody prepares us to get old; we aren't ready for it. So many of us have incomes so low they don't even reach the subsistence level."

"But I don't like being old."

"It could be worse for you if you were black or Mexican American. Chances are you'd be much poorer and in bad health too. Since we live in the city, we probably have a lower status than the old folks in the country. Now, tell me where your sisters are."

"At the Ball. I must clean the kitchen before they return."

"Why aren't you going to the Ball? That makes me furious!" Her small wrinkled face contorted with anger. "Tell me what you want. Do you want to go to the Ball?"

"I used to be a good dancer, but they told me I'm too old now, nobody would want to dance with me. And they're right."

The little woman drew herself up to full height. "You're going. And wait and see. You'll have a wonderful time. I know."

Cinderella brushed her fine white hair up into a knot and quickly washed the dust from her face.

"Do I look okay?" she asked as she turned around. But the little woman was gone.

The Prince had always given an appearance of youthfulness,

but up close the sisters could see that he was no longer a
young man. He was a regal figure, and as handsome as they
had anticipated. Bula's eagerness overcame her, and she pushed through the crowd to him almost knocking guests over in
her haste. Not to be outdone, the other sisters followed closely.

"Sign my dance card, Prince Charming," breathed Bula.
She gave her sisters a triumphant look as the Prince took out
his pen. "Oh, sign more than once..."

"My dear, I must do my duty by the others as well," he
answered hurriedly, hoping to escape. As he looked at the
others he realized he would be no better off with them. He
signed all the cards dejectedly.

"Look!" cried Jaypea. Cinderella walked through the door
proudly. She appeared taller now, and no longer shuffled
along dragging her feet. "Is it really Cinderella?"

"It is! I told her to stay home." said Hippocrata. "You
heard me, didn't you Bula?"

"She looks like an old crazy woman standing over there.
She probably doesn't know where she is!"

But she didn't look crazy to the Prince, as he looked to
see what was causing such an uproar. The frail delicate woman interested him immediately. Her simple dress made her
stand out among the gaudily dressed women. He began to
make his way toward her. But the music started, and Bula
grabbed his arm possessively, fluttering her eyelashes.

"It's our dance, Prince," she said. He could hardly reach
around her as he worried she would crush his toes. She pressed closer until she could whisper in his ear, "Whatever you
want, I'm ready to give you."

"I do want something of you, Bula." Her mouth dropped
surprise making a row of chins upon her neck.

"I heard what you said about Cinderella and..."

"But,"

"Listen to me, you selfish woman. Don't you see what you
are doing to her? Look at your fine dress, then look at her
rags. Look at your indulgent fat, then look how thin she is."

"But she is old and ugly. She doesn't need new clothes.
And why should we waste our food on her?"

"To me she is a beautiful person with much to offer."

"She is a pain," Bula wailed. "Always asking for more
money!"

"I want you to change. For me, and all old people."

She nodded miserably as the dance ended.

Again Prince Charming began to go to Cinderella, but a
cold strong hand stopped him. He turned to look into the
sunning shrewd eyes of Jaypea.

"Oh, hello," he said. "What a beautiful dress. And did
you go to the hairdresser's?"

"Thank you, Prince Charming. I spent hours at the hairdresser's and shopped for my dress for days. Just for you."

"And what did Cinderella do while you were shopping? Why
doesn't she have a new dress? And fancy curls in her hair?"

Jaypea turned white with rage. "She is old and useless. I
want her out of the house. She slows things down. If we didn't
have her, we could hire someone young and efficient to do our
cleaning. Someone who didn't break dishes, who could manage
money."

"You are a cruel woman. I don't want to believe you are
that cold all the way through. Cinderella needs self-esteem
and self-respect. You have taken that away from her. Make
her feel wanted and needed once again."

Jaypea reluctantly let go as the music stopped. Dulce was
waiting nearby and grabbed the Prince's hand.

"Do these musicians ever take a break?" asked the Prince
in despair, as he glanced over the crowd to find Cinderella.

"Perhaps they will after our dance and we can stroll out
to the balcony where we can be alone. Oh, I've waited so
long for this mement."

"I have waited a long time too, but only to ask you why
you pretend to love your stepsister when you really don't
like her?"

"But I don't pretend, I do love her, anyone can see that,"
she said sweetly.

"Then why do you treat her as a child? Why don't you let
her make her own decisions instead of making them for her?"

"How do you know what I do?"

"It is my business to know what happens in the Kingdom.
Ask her if she wants to live with you. Ask her what she
wants for her life. Then perhaps you won't feel so guilty and
angry about her."

He left Dulce in the center of the dance floor as the music
stopped. but Hippocrata wasn't easily eluded.

"Did you forget our dance? After all the time "I've waited
for you?"

By now Prince Charming was beginning to lose his temper
with these women.

"I suppose you primped all day and rested while Cinderella
scrubbed the floors."

"Why do you want to talk about an old senile woman? She
ought to be put away. She forgets where she is. I don't
want to try to help her anymore. I don't understand her and
I don't want to *try* to understand her."

"Why should she have to struggle to get enough to eat and
stay alive when you don't have to? Her life shouldn't be any
more difficult than yours."

The dance finally ended and the Prince found Cinderella.
He noticed how the lights reflected silver from her hair.

"I would be honored to have this dance, Cinderella."

She could hardly believe it. Only an hour ago she had
been scrubbing pots and pans, and now she was in Prince
Charming's arms. Out of the corner of her eyes, she could
see her stepsisters watching with envy as one dance ended and
another began. Still the Prince danced on.

"I want to show you something. Look over there."

She saw an elderly man giving orders to all the waiters
and waitresses. "He is the manager of that department, and
a good one. His experience throughout the years is invaluable
to us. It is difficult for older people to find jobs when we have
to compete with younger workers. Technology changes so rapidly
that many times our skills are outdated. Do you miss your old
job?"

Before she could answer he whirled her around to the other
side of the ballroom, where she saw a woman living happily in a
nursing home, content to be with others her age. Another woman kept her grandchildren content while the daughter prepared

supper. Yet another man lived all alone, but savored his
independence.

"What I'm trying to show you, Cinderella, is that you can
do whatever you want here. It is all here, waiting for you.
Tell me now, what will make you happy?"

But then, the clock struck twelve.

Psychiatry as it relates to the elderly is mired in crises today.
But to appreciate Psychiatry's crisis, one must first be aware of the
issues faced daily by the elderly.

The allegory helps to depict certain key aspects of their problems,
as portrayed by the plight of Cinderella. It can be seen from the not-so-
incredible fairy tale that the plight of the elderly is made considerably
more difficult, if not caused, by obstacles blocking their paths during
the later and late portions of the life cycle. Many of these obstacles are
created by major unavoidable forces impacting upon the elderly. In the
fairy tale, the obstacles were portrayed by the stepsisters. Jaypea
represents Commerce; Hippocrata, Medicine; Bulacratta, Government; and
Dulce, Family. Singularly, or in concert, these forces may overwhelm
even the most stable individual and produce dysfunction, including mental
illness. Psychiatry's crisis lies in the fact that the mental health care
needs of the aged are being met poorly, and little hope exists for future
improvement unless changes are made.

COMMERCE

Perhaps business and industry have the earliest impact on the aging
and aged. Probably the most negative intersection of commerce with
the elderly has occurred in the employment arena.

In 1870, 70 percent of the aged were gainfully employed. In contrast,
only 20 percent of the men age 65 and older and 8 percent of the women
age 65 and older were in the U.S. labor force in 1977. These figures
persist despite the fact that 95 percent of the U.S. elderly are not
institutionalized, and 85 percent are ambulatory and functional for some
form of employment. In 1975, unemployment among those 45 years and
older was the highest in the nation's history, increasing by 28 percent
over the preceding ten years. Further, the duration of unemployment
is longer for older workers when compared to younger populations. In
1975, the average length of joblessness for a 45-54-year-old worker was
15.8 weeks; for those 55-64, 17.8 weeks; and for those 65 and older, six
months. Retirement is the principal reason for the elderly's absence
from the labor market. And it is occurring at progressively younger
ages. Unfortunately, it has been estimated that 40 percent of all retirees
cease work involuntarily.

The major adverse effects of retirement are those resulting from
loss. Financially, a sharp drop in income occurs. As life expectancy
increases, people live a progressively greater number of years without
employment – often in poverty. Projections show that out of every 100
persons starting financially "even" at age 25, 1 will be rich in 40 years,
4 independent, 5 having to work, 36 dead, and 54 dependent on another
person or an agency for monetary support. Regardless of the size of
income at the time of retirement, maintenance of an adequate income
throughout old age is a problem for most Americans. At any time the
median income of this population is considerably less than that of their
younger counterparts. In 1975, families headed by a person 65 years
or older had a median income of $8,057, compared with $14,698 for
younger family units. In 1977, one-sixth of all elderly persons lived

in households with annual incomes below the official poverty level
($3,417 for older couples and $2,720 for older individuals.)   Chances
of being poor are 50 percent greater if one is 65 years or older.   Certain subgroups among the elderly emerge as relatively more disadvantaged than others.   For example, elderly blacks have one-third less
income than whites.   Elderly females have one-half the median income
of elderly males.   The poorest of the poor are black aged females living alone, approximately two-thirds of whom are classified as "poor"
and 78 percent, "very poor."

HEALTH

Health problems arise in the lives of the aging and aged perhaps
as often as problems of early retirement and poverty.   Seventy-two
percent of those in the middle years and 86 percent of the geriatric
population have one chronic illness.   Fifty percent of the elderly have
two or more chronic illnesses.

Medical care of aged patients in the United States has been alleged
to be characerized by negativism, defeatism, and professional antipathy.
This is manifested most commonly as a therapeutic nihilism toward their
treatment.   The credo of clinical practice with the elderly has been
based all to frequently on the false premise that since old age is irreversible, illness occurring in late life likewise must be irreversible.

Palliation and psychopharmacological "control," with little regard
for remission and optimal rehabilitation, frequently constitute the main-
stays of treatment.   Physicians and other health care professionals
often omnisciently and omnipotently determine the quality of life that
they believe someone 65 years or older deserves, solely by age.   Commonly, the assumption is made regardless of the patient's desires.

Negative attitudes toward aging and the aged are believed to account
in great part for such care.   Apart from the elderly's qualitatively and
quantitatively deficient care, negative attitudes also may be noted in
the utterances of medical students, housestaff, and faculty.   Examples
include "over-the-hill," "hopeless," "crock," "gomer," "toad," "nursing
home dump," and "dirtball."   Medical students' prejudice against the
elderly has been observed to be stronger than prejudice against color.
Faculty attitudes influence those of their students.   One study revealed
that medical students' attitudes toward aging and the aged actually de-
teriorated over their four-year curriculum.   Recent studies have demonstrated educator negativism to surpass that of the students.

Such attitudes may be subsumed under the term "ageism," defined
as a bias against the old merely because of their age.   Threats to
immortality, reawakened parental conflicts, self-perceived clinical in-
competence, and feelings of low prestige prompted by exposure to the
elderly are a few common causal conditions.   Health provider discomfort
precipitated by these factors tends to produce avoidance of the elderly
and their problems.

GOVERNMENT

Government has now assumed the primary role in allocation of financial assistance to the elderly, in the form of retirement support and
health care insurance.   However, the responsibility for the financial
care of the elderly once lay with the family, and those without families
were taken to county institutions.

In 1883, California made grants to counties with families who attempted maintenance of the aged in their homes, as well as to those who

gave out relief. Because of abuses, however, these programs were
discontinued in 1895. Monetary contributions then went to state-level
institutions only.

After examination of the plight of its elderly in 1929, California
adopted a law extending relief to all needy old people. This action
paved the way for other action, and by 1934 thirty states had some
form of assistance program. In addition, philanthropists, trade unions,
and churches had begun to build old folks' homes.

In 1935, the federal government became more directly involved by
the passage of the Social Security Act. This legislation provided a
type of insurance with future benefits based directly on cumulative
contributions made by individuals during their work lives. It also
authorized federal grants to those states that provided programs of aid
to the aged. Amendments in 1939 altered this to include spouse benefits, a progressive benefits formula, a minimum benefit, and a work
text. By 1943, 23.4 percent of the U.S. aged received some form of
financial aid, but only 3.4 percent received retirement pensions.

In 1951, the immense majority of the elderly still had incomes far
below the subsistence level. Although the number of those benefitting
from Social Security gradually increased, the incomes of 25 percent of
elderly couples and 50 percent of elderly single women had not reached
subsistence levels in 1975.

The 1960s witnessed an increase in legislative activity concerning
social and health concerns. As part of the governmental impetus, the
Older Americans Act, and Title XVIII (Medicare) and Title XIV (Medicaid) of the Social Security Act were passed in 1965. But 15 years
later, the rate of poverty among the elderly is approximately twice that
of younger populations.

In 1976, per capita health care costs of the elderly came to $1,521,
or 3.5 times the $438 spent for each individual younger than 65. Most
of the money spent was in relation to chronic illnesses. The elderly's
share of these expenses continues to increase and, currently, it is
the highest it has ever been. Average older Americans spent $613 of
their own money for medical services during 1977, or 35 percent of
their total health care bill. During that same year, Medicare covered
only approximately 41 percent of aged Americans' total health care
expenditures nationwide. State Medicaid programs paid an additional
16.7 percent. Despite the fact that the most commonly reported chronic
illnesses of the elderly are hearing and visual impairments, as well as
arthritis, Medicare does not cover eye glasses, hearing aids, or podia-
tric care. Furthermore, prescriptions and over-the-counter medications
represent approximately 50 percent of the elderly's health care expenditures. Yet Medicare does not reimburse the elderly for these commodities.
Medicaid will not reimburse the elderly for nursing home care unless
that individual is taking medication!

FAMILY

In the early part of this century, American society was almost
totally oriented toward bringing people into a family system and maintaining them there. The latter part of the life cycle was expected to
be, more or less, a continuation of the middle years. The nuclear and
extended family served as a setting for this transition.

But society, as well as the family, has gradually turned away from
the aged since World War II — especially from older women. One-third
of them live alone, as opposed to the 80 percent of men who live in a
family setting. Fortunately, many of those living alone continue to

maintain some form of contact with family.

However, contact with families is not always anxiety-free for either the elderly individual or the younger family member(s). Difficulties may arise from conflict between the agendas of each age camp. These conflicts have great potential consequences for the old person, often dependent on his or her family for support of one form or another. The most unfortunate consequence, should conflicts not be reconciled, is extrusion. Alternative sources of gratification are usually suboptimal when compared with the significance of families.

To more fully appreciate sources of conflict, a review of some commonly noted "agendas" often acted out in the family setting is helpful. Many elderly are maintained in the home for fear of religious retribution. Others are maintained so that the younger individuals can satisfy previously ungratified needs to be a "better" son or daughter. Of course, they may do so to capitalized on the elder's estate.

The aged person may also be "used" as a "convenient" wedge between the younger couple to prevent contact in an already troubled marriage. It would be unfair to shift blame to younger persons alone, however, since the elderly individual in most cases has the capacity to accept or decline the invitation to "move in" or "remain" in the children's home. Further, the aged person likewise has an agenda that he may seek to fulfill in the family setting. Several frequently observed elderly persons' agendas include: a need to complete the unfinished business of being a "better" parent; feeling of helplessness resulting from the need to fend for oneself; a desire to control family members when other more usual sources for control are no longer available; and a role to feel useful by performing usual and previously done household tasks.

THE PROBLEM AND THE CRISIS

Each of these forces creates a potential stress on the elderly individual. These occur at a time of progressively declining reserves to withstand such stresses, and with a prolonged recuperation period to pre-stress baseline.

Utilizing the model of homeostasis, it is not difficult to appreciate the increased risk of disequilibrium (and consequent disease) as one grows older. Actual age-related homeostatic disruption is borne out by illness statistics of the late-life population, which depict a rising incidence of psychopathology with advancement through the life cycle. Compare the following figures: The incidence of mental illness in persons 15 years of age and younger has been reported at 2.3 cases per 100,000. This is in sharp contrast to 236.1 cases per 100,000 in persons 65 years of age and older. Currently, approximately $2\frac{1}{2}$ to $5\frac{1}{2}$ million U.S. elderly have some form of pyschiatric illness requiring therapeutic intervention.

Although corrective measures have been set in motion, the crisis facing American Psychiatry is that the mental health needs of 80 to 93 percent of the psychiatrically ill elderly are not met through existing resources. U.S. psychiatrists spend less than two percent of their time treating the elderly, and no greater than four percent of the elderly are seen in community mental health facilities. In addition, most nursing homes (60 to 70 percent of whose residents have psychiatric illness) are without ongoing psychiatric services. Since the geriatric age group is the fastest growing segment of our population, this problem will worsen as the years pass.

The crisis continues. Of those elderly who do have access to psychiatric services, most receive qualitatively suboptimal care. A therapuetic nihilism often pervails with respect to their treatment. Use of psychopharmacologics for palliation and control frequently replaces thoughtful and careful attempts at remission and reapproximation of the individual's pre-morbid baseline. For example, seventy-five percent of nursing home residents receive one or more psychotropic medications. In the face of age-related declines in physiological reserves, however, the risk of medication-induced iatrogenic disease rises. This rate has been observed to be 23 percent in the 70 to 79 age groups, as opposed to 3 percent in the 20 to 29 age group. Contributing to such unnecessary iatrogenic illness are other factors: inadequate diagnostic assessment (inferential, rather than a scrutinizing and comprehensive examination); non-indicated drug prescription; suboptimal dosage regimens (including inappropriately high or low dosages, without remission as an endpoint); inadequate prepsychopharmacologic physiological evaluation; and poor followup psychiatric assessment both to determine the need for regimen changes and to monitor for the appearance of significant side effects.

Suboptimal psychiatric care assumes many other forms as well. Incomplete and noncomprehensive assessment often precludes adequate treatment dispositions. Such assessments frequently do not include the perspectives of those disciplines that impact on the patient's past, present, and future. Assessment is usually vague, impersonal, and superficial. Frequently, it is made by telephone, with treatment rendered on the basis of input from someone other than the psychiatric physician. Goals of rehabilitation and optimal therapy are not employed. Pre-morbid assessment in basic life areas (which represent the activity sought by the patient to maintain psychological comfort) are not considered. These baseline areas include preferences in interpersonal relationships, work, education, nutrition, religion, recreation, personality, and so on. Without this, health care professionals do not have a reasonable point to which they can return the patient or even reapproximate. Absence of such assessment means no indications are made of which psychosocial therapies would create iatrogenic stresses; for example, the basically introverted individual does not wish to "boogie". This is indicative of fitting the patient to the treatment as opposed to individualizing treatment for the elderly patient. Too often, when one becomes 65, it is auto- matically assumed that the individual has an overwhelming desire to make potholders and ashtrays, tool leather belts, and/or beat tambourines!

Additionally, hospital stays tend to be short. Frequently, an old person's condition is assessed as "just senility." This implies irreversi- bility and, therefore, attempts at etiological detection and reversal are not made. Attempts at remission do not ensue. It is all too commonly assumed that something magical happens between ages 64 and 65 making mental illness in late life beyond significant assistance.

Normal states also are often "treated" to maintain the quiescence of the health care personnel. One study revealed that many old persons feel it is vitally important to be heard. Some have said that arguing keeps them warm and lets them know they are still alive. Many may wish to recount the past. And yet, such behavior may be poorly tolerated and frequently results in a call to the doctor for pharmacological treatment and extrusion from existing settings. For example, an elderly individual often has no selection privileges. He may have to eat his evening meal at 4:30 in the afternoon, have fried chicken or spinach, when he doesn't like it, and so on. Attempts at change may meet with resistence. Perhaps equally as serious is the situation in which the elderly individual, dependent on family or institution for sustenance, wishes to voice his or her legitimate feelings but cannot, for fear of extrusion or retribution.

Another issue in the elderly's care is their right to refuse treatment.

Few attempts are made to explain treatment to them, and they do not
have ample opportunity to voice their feelings about it. It is as if they
yield this right when they become 65. This may breed noncompliance,
especially in the presence of side effects.

Regardless of the reasons for the physician's, other health care
professional's, or society's negative attitudes, they are often obvious
or can be inferred by many elderly. Their prevalence can be overwhelming, causing the aged individual to believe them. In some, this
posture may coincide with personality style. That is, the person may
be ready to submit and gain psychological comfort and, much the same
as our Cinderella, may actually accept such treatment as his lot in life.
Unfortunately, the elderly may actually begin to devalue themselves in
the process. Those who fight it may meet with failure–additional confirmation of their "cloutless" status. For those not yet willing to be
seen as hopeless and beyond help or attention, it is a true tragic waste
of human life. Change or circumvention become more difficult with
rising age, as alternatives tend to decrease.

A RESPONSE TO THE PRESENT

And so appears the fairy Godmother to shake Cinderella loose from
myths about herself, giving her an opportunity to gain more from her
future. She speaks to and for Cinderella. She tells of the inequalities
that many aged suffer–and how she herself has suffered them. Perhaps
she tells Cinderella many things.

For example, nothing "magical" happens during the night a person
is age 64 and the next morning, when he becomes 65. Old age does not
happen at 65; a person has been aging since shortly after conception.
Therefore, the 65th birthday is merely a point in a continuum that
begins with birth and ends with death. At age 65, the elderly individual
presents with a past, present, and presumably a future. The past is
a compilation of the means by which the patient sought to maintain
psychological homeostasis. The present quite possibly represents a
situation in which stresses impinging on the individual have exceeded the
defenses mustered against those stresses. The future will be much like
the pre-morbid past, in terms of the individual's perceptions of life
events and the quality/quantity of his or her responses. However, in
most cases it will be marked by lowered physiological and psychological
reserves to withstand stress; a qualitative and quantitative increase
in stress; and a slower return to pre-stress baseline. In addition, the
future will be marked by the fact that it is the last stage of life–a factor
that separates this stage of the life cycle from the balance. Because
of the significance of this finality, many elderly feel it is incumbent
upon them to get their lives in order, so that death may be preceeded
by a sense of relative psychological equanimity and calm. To accomplish
this, they often take a retrospective journey through their lives–recalling
their pasts–to gain satisfaction from personally rewarding life events
and to gain perspective on the less gratifying ones. During this life
review, it is helpful to the elderly person to have interested people
around to lend support to his plight. Once life's deficits are established,
the individual may embark on a course of restitution in an attempt to
gain psychological homeostasis. The success with which this life review
is accomplished depends upon several factors, some of which are summarized as follows:
1. The degree of "unfinished business" the individual finds on retro-
spection and introspection. In essence, a longer list in the light of
limited time can become potentially overwhelming.

2.   The success with which a person has tolerated stress in the preceding years.
3.   The ability to sublimate.
4.   The willingness of key segments of the individual's environment to permit gratification of sublimatory outlets.
    The fairy Godmother would tell Cinderella for all to hear:
    —That both onset, and rate and quality of aging are individual issues defying generalization.
    —That diseases in late life are not different from those in younger years, although prevalence rates may change.
    —That outcome of mental illness treatment of reversible states should not be significantly different for the elderly.
    —That poor technique, including psychopharmacological technique in younger years, will probably find its way to the geriatric patient with potentially more severe outcome.
    —That optimal technique for the treatment of psychiatric disease includes compliance with several important requirements: (1) Treatment must assist the individual to fulfill certain needs, such as the desire to gain satisfaction from life thus far.   (2) Restoration of balance must be achieved, and since nonpsychiatric illness may be an etiological factor, a comprehensive physiological evaluation should be done.   (3) A multidisciplinary team is the key to treatment of the elderly because key areas from a patient's past, present, and future need to be considered. (4) Optimal treatment requires sufficient time for remission of a reversible state, and preparation of the postdischarge receiving environment. (5) Strategies and dosages must be adjusted to meet age and physiological needs.   (6) And, last, therapeutic plans must be individualized.
    —That neither the physician nor other health care providers have the right to decide what the individual's quality of life should be like, but that they do have an obligation to offer every opportunity for a healthy, productive, and happy life.
    —That a large body of knowledge is available on care of the geriatric patient.   It needs to be not only disseminated but enlarged.

THE FUTURE

    In our fairy tale, the Prince holds the key to exposing Cinderella to a potentially rewarding future!   The stepsisters continue in their efforts to sabotage the attempts of the Prince to do so.   Despite this, Cinderella gains a glimpse of what might be.
    For example, she sees an elderly person employed in a setting that discriminates only on the basis of ability and not age.   A setting in which permission to work beyond the usual retirement age is not accompanied by humiliation, reductions in responsibilities, salary, and quality of work settings.
    She sees several settings that were selected by the elderly—not health care providers, in the absence of assessment and input from the elderly.   She sees that these health care providers no longer assume omnipotence and omnisicience in the rendering of these decisions, that they accept the individuality of aging and assist in making decisions accordingly.
    Were Cinderella to look further into the future, she would see other positive trends afoot in the United States.   She would see more health professions schools beginning to add gerontology (science of aging) and geriatrics (diseases of the aged) to the curricula.   She would realize that not everyone in Commerce, Health, Government, and Family feels negatively toward aging and the aged.   And she would see the beginning

of more positive attitudes emerging among those who had been negative. These attitudes would clarify previously held myths about aging and the aged.

She would see a growing awareness among scientists, clinicians, and lay persons that problems with memory and cognition do not represent "normal" aging. When memory problems do occur, they represent pathology requiring etiological evaluation—10 to 30 percent of organic brain syndromes in late life have potentially reversible etiologies if evaluated and treated in time. She would find that the term "senility" is representative of ageism and does not represent any pathological state per se. It serves only as a justification for lack of therapeutic interventions among the disinterested. She would find that reversible states have as much potential for reversal in late life as in younger years. She would see that optimal health technique for illness in late life requires a sound working knowledge of the particular field-at-large, with the application of special age-related nuances. She would see the major goal of health care as the production of remission, vigorous attempts to return the patient to pre-morbid baseline, and maintenance of the improved state.

Among the other myths and stereotypes beginning to be dispelled is that regarding the uniformity of aging. Specifically, not everyone ages in the same way and at the same rate. Chronological age often is an inaccurate prediction of physical, mental, and emotional status. The myth of unproductivity also needs to be scrutinized more carefully. Again, it is an individual matter. The capacity for some form of gainful employment can continue as long as the individual wishes. Reduction to a disabled state generally stems from the minds and hearts of younger segments of society.

The myth of the "suffering old" will be discredited. All aged do not suffer, despite loss. Their capacity to rebound and perceive their environment are functions of reactions in younger years. All too frequently, the eyes of the observer pattern perceptions of the old. The observer must see through the eyes of the elderly to make more accurate perceptions. Finally, the tendency of society to segregate and sequester groups from the mainstream will begin to decline.

Society will begin to see its older populace as individuals, and not purely as ages. Society must, because the clock is striking twelve.

REFERENCES

Butler, R.N. *Why Survive? Being Old in America*. New York: Harper and Row, Publishers, 1975.

Butler, R.N. Clinical psychiatry in late life. In *Clinical Geriatrics*, Rossman, I. (ed.). Philadelphia: J.B. Lippincott, 1971, pp. 439-459.

Cohen, G.D. Mental health services and the elderly: Needs and options. *Am. J. Psychiat.* 133:65, 1976.

Levenson, A.J. Preferences in gerontologic and geriatrics training in medical school: A Comparison of medical students, educators, and general practitioners. *J. Am. Ger. Soc.* (in press).

Levenson, A.J. (ed.). *Neuropsychiatric Side Effects of Drugs in the Elderly*. New York: Raven Press, 1979.

Levenson, A.J. and Felkins, B.J. Prevention of psychiatric recidivism: A Model Service. *J. Am. Ger. Soc.* 17:536, 1979.

Levenson, A.J.; Cohen, G.D.; Gershell, W.J.; Hall, R.C.W.; and Finkel, S.I. Geriatric psychopharmacotherapy: Optimal technique. In *Proceedings of 32nd Annual Scientific Meeting of Gerontological*

Society. Washington, D.C., November 1979.
Task panel reports submitted to the President's Commission on Mental
   Health.   3:Appendix.   Washington, D.C.: U.S. Government
   Printing Office, 1978.
Weinberg, J.   Geriatric psychiatry.   In *Comprehensive Textbook of
   Psychiatry II*, Freedman, A.; Kaplan, H.; Sadock, B. (eds.).
   Baltimore: Williams and Wilkins Co., 1975).

14

The Social Role of Psychiatry: A Look Forward to the Eighties

Chester M. Pierce

INTRODUCTION

As we enter the eighties, social psychiatry must look forward to crises and changes. Before discussing such crises and changes, some definitions must be established. The substance of these definitions embraces every life and regards matters that influence every life. The context in which these projections are made is guided by the overwhelming reality of the world-wide tensions stemming from energy problems and consequent economic stress in the United States. How American people respond to these crises and changes between now and 1990 will influence the emotional and mental life of everyone on earth.

In this sense, the crises truly represent opportunities and challenges. A major change for the mental health worker in the United States may be the necessity to be more occupied by dysfunctions of entitlement (Pierce, 1978). The basic characteristic of entitlement dysfunctions are perceptual differences among communicants in regard to rights, duties, privileges, or obligations. The perceptual differences involve interpersonal confrontations in which prestige/status conflicts are more salient and expressive than frustrations or obstacles involving sex, dependency, or aggression. Clinically, the issues describe considerations of hegemony about the disrepectful and undignified use, misuse, or abuse of someone's time, space, energy, and mobilization.

Overall, the pressures dictated by the harsh economic realities and ever-increasing burdens to the environment demand that a primary concern must be to move all people to the status of planetary citizens. To reach the status of a cosmopolitan society, all citizens in the United States may have to aspire to relatively less, and possess relatively less, than citizens elsewhere. Such a situation should be anticipated to cause stressful sociopolitical and cultural problems that will bring about ongoing and numberless entitlement dysfunctions in Americana.

Therefore, the resolution of entitlement dysfunctions represents the opportunity and challenge for social psychiatry in the 1980s. A leading textbook defines social psychiatry as that branch of psychiatry "interested in ecological, sociological, and cultural variables that engender, intensify, or complicate maladaptive patterns of behavior and their treatment" (Freedman, Kaplan and Sadock, 1975).

Such a definition charges social psychiatry with a near limitless concern. Therefore, the social psychiatrist is obliged to consider submolecular to macromolecular forms that interfere with human adjustment. The scope of concern is complicated by unforeseen circumstances, such as inventions, pestilence, war or famine, as they mold behavior of individuals or masses. In practice, no fine lines exist between what is adaptive and what is nonadaptive; what is cause and what is effect; what is science and what is research.

Hence, the theoretical predictions of the eighties have the quality of balancing what is and what should be, in the same sense that the clinician balances these aspects of the art in everyday practice.

Based on present trends, the social psychiatrist, in his struggle against entitlement dysfunctions, will be working: (1) in much closer alliance with medicine, medical practitioners, and the medical model, and (2) to effect more benefits to patients via preventive and prophylactic techniques.

With this as an introduction, the bulk of the chapter will deal with specifying several major crises of social psychiatry and presenting possible routes to maximize the opportunities presented by the crises. As in many life situations, the crises overlap, and both support and inform one another. Hence, the solutions require a much more integrated and comprehensive approach than what is outlined in only a conspectus.

THE ECOLOGICAL CRISIS: CAN WE CONTROL CLIMATES?

Significantly, the first portion of the definition of the field of social psychiatry speaks of ecology. In the broadest way, all human behavior and emotions in the 1980s depend on global response to the decrease in productive crop lands, increase in urban sprawl, and increase in desert-ification secondary to deforestations, overgrazing, and overplowing of land. The contribution of the social psychiatrist to remediation of these ills, mediated often by unregulated or poorly regulated technology, is paradoxically insignificant but important. The social psychiatrist must be one of a plethora of contributors who work in systems analysis to insure and preserve better living and working environments.

To meet this crisis the social psychiatrist of the 1980s is challenged to become more involved in research, especially about problems of fear and violence. In collaboration with social and physical scientists, social psychiatrists should be concerned about efforts to effectively control the natural as well as artificial environments. Of course, this is not a new interest for social psychiatrists, since even in the tenth century A.D., in the anonymous Paradise of Wisdom, physicians reorganized the temperamental differences in men from the deserts as compared with men of the sea.

However, given the social context to the beginning of the 1980s fear and violence must be investigated and collated with research in other disciplines. For instance, despite the rigors of the economy, people feel entitled not only to a job, but also to a good job. At the same time, people continue to want shorter work weeks, but do more part-time work. By May 1977, 4.6 million people held two or more jobs (Best, 1978).

What is germane to the social psychiatrist who struggles with maladaptation, is that more people are unsuited for their jobs and are dissatisfied and discontent. Therefore, despite not inconsiderable unemployment or underemployment, many people express less interest in their work, and make less effort on their jobs. U.S. Bureau of Labor Statistics data indicate that work may have absorbed one-third of an average person's life span in primitive times. Today, an American male works less than 13% of his life.

Meanwhile, on the one hand, many jobs have excessive educational requirements. On the other hand, lower grade jobs are unfilled because everyone feels entitled to more prestigious, psychologically satisfying work. The fears from mounting economic insecurity are at seeming variance with many attitudes of people about work and their job climates. If social stability requires more people to do with less and to work in even less satisfying job climates, violence can be anticipated.

New views about jobs may involve more social psychiatrists. Recently, a policeman was successful in getting compensation for the stress occasioned by his work as a patrolman. He cited the fact that the conditions encountered on his job required him to seek psychiatric treatment. Another case pending involves a group of black men who claim that racial discrimination encountered in their blue collar jobs caused them irreparable damage. Depending on one's perception of entitlements, one can argue whether a patrolman's beat does more damage to someone than racial discrimination. No matter what one perceives, however, surely someone else will perceive differently. In the 1980s, these perceptions of who's entitled to what living, work, or educational space may promote increasing fears and violence.

Yet, as Eisenberg points out, there will be relatively fewer psychiatrists (Eisenberg, 1979). Further, those psychiatrists who practice may have relatively less interest or inclination to "social psychiatry" as opposed to more "biological psychiatry." This emphasizes the need for fundamental research to be directed on fear and violence. A special part of this research should be toward producing information that could be disseminated and used by primary care physicians, as they labor with increasing numbers of patients whose entitlement dysfunctions move them to more fearful and/or violent attitudes and behavior. Such attitudes and behavior not only make for turbulent life styles but, in fact, may contribute to physical illness, as well as, of course, accidents.

Other sorts of artificial environments could be cited that need to be controlled and that could profit from fundamental research on fear and violence as they relate to systems and individual psychopathology. For instance, cities are densely clustered populations competing for increasingly scarce resources. In such a background, unruly crowds at sports events, neighborhood anger about airplane noise intrusion, civic waste, or community resistance to a proposed adjacent housing project, all bespeak of common sites for fear and violence in urban areas. The urban climate must be controlled in order to sustain sufficient ecological tranquility to allow humans not to "engender, intensify, or complicate maladaptive patterns of behavior."

For a variety of reasons, society has elected to give over more study to preparing for and managing disasters. The input of research by social psychiatrists interested in systems could yield positive spin-off results that would aid urban ecology. Thus, in studying fear and violence as they relate to earthquakes, nuclear disasters, fires, floods, hurricanes, or terrorists' acts, there will be insights that could help urban existence by telling a bit more about how more people can live longer, better, and together.

Lastly, in terms of the ecological crisis and the need for systems integration of research on violence and fear, there is an area few psychiatrists recognize as important to their inquiries. This area is the area of natural climate control. Since January 1, 1979, dozens of countries all over the world have been involved in a collaborative research program, designed over a twenty-five year period, for the purpose of weather modification. The immediate step is directed toward more long-range weather forecasting. However, an intermediate step,

at an indefinite future date, will have as its goal some weather modification. Ultimately, there is hope that some considerable degree of
climate control will be achieved (Climate Research Board, 1978; Global
Atmospheric Research Program, 1977). The consequences of this
experiment, if successful, will be mind-boggling in terms of food
production, transportation, communication, and development of technology.
It seems not excessive to say that over the course of the next fifty
years, data analyzed and experiments begun in the 1980s may indeed
influence all aspects of existence, both animate and inanimate.

As with any important or massive scientific advance such as the
development of printing or atomic energy or computers, posterity is
committed and people begin to feel, think, and behave differently.
For these reasons, the Global Atmospheric Research Program, which
has been "done quietly" as "an audacious venture, unprecedented in
terms of cooperative, international, scientific endeavor," will have
increasing, if subtle, impact in the 1980s, (U.S. Com. for the Global
Atmospheric Research Program, 1978). Predictably, many thoughtful
people will have concerns as they become aware of such experiments.
Many issues will have to be debated. The social psychiatrists should
be involved in the research on the effects of possible climate control on
human systems. Doubtlessly, many people will be fearful and angry
about experiments of this sort, whether or not they have any degree
of technical understanding of the goals. People may become violent
as a result of awareness of attempts to control the weather. Nearly
everyone will have some fear and trepidation as humans take a quantum
leap to control their surroundings.

THE SOCIOLOGICAL CRISIS: CAN WE CONTAIN COSTS?

The essence of the definition of sociology is, "How do aggregates
of humans act?" As such, the sociological crisis to be addressed must
consider the forms, functions, and effects of aggregations of humans
at the outset of the 1980s. Inflation is a major problem for most human
groups. During the 1980s the social psychiatrists need to add expertise
to the problem of containing costs. One way this can be accomplished
is through the help of the social psychiatrist in making delivery of
health care more cost-effective.

If costs are not contained whole populations will be stressed, and
disharmony, the mate to strife, will hold sway. Several means to reduce
health costs can be delineated.

As mentioned earlier, the relative dearth of psychiatrists renders
it obligatory that primary care physicians do much therapeutic and
preventive mental health work. This means that close, meaningful
interactions between psychiatrists and primary care physicians must be
nurtured and maintained. A principal location for such interaction
would be any medical setting where psychiatrists serve as consultants
or liaison physicians. During the 1980s, the liaison-consultant
psychiatrists will have to be more cost-conscious, as collaboration
proceeds with other doctors in an effort to anticipate and dilute or
prevent mental distress and disease.

Second, the social psychiatrists will have to bring these same
attitudes of preventive care to community sites. Whenever working with
neighborhood organizations, self-help groups, or community agencies,
the doctor will have to be mindful that increased expenditures, particularly for curative medicine, do not bring about an automatic increased
effectiveness of treatment. In fact, an investigator writing in the
early 1970s could lament that, despite greatly increased quantities of

resources allocated for medical care, in the two previous decades there had been a parallel decline in the mortality rate to virtually zero (Powles, 1972).

Perhaps the expanded preventive approach in the 1980s will require that social psychiatrists employ more manipulation of demographics. It may be time to develop mental health checkups that can be administered easily to large populations, such as factory and office workers, or to farmers or transportation workers.

Indeed, in some areas of occupational psychiatry, theories and tools have been developed that might be applied to many other groups in the quest for means of accomplishing mass mental checkups. Arthur (1971) has summarized studies by the military to predict vocational success. Basically, it is possible to combine empirically derived quantitative data to screen and select individuals for tasks. The prediction methods of the 1980s could make use of relatively static or unchanging information (age, sex, race, schooling, intelligence, family stability, legal infractions) and temporary or transient data (recent life events, leadership or followership situations, task satisfaction). This material, combined with selective physiological and biochemical data, could be used to compute the chances for emotional turmoil, as well as to illuminate potential areas of difficulty.

To establish an early warning system in itself could require monumental expense and administration. However, the data accumulated could be used to make even more refined predictions. Further, without some rather large-scale efforts at this sort of preventive service delivery, no meaningful system of mental health checkups can be developed. One could visualize that service delivery by 1990 would make use of periodic checkups, perhaps largely administered by nonphysicians. The doctor could then take computerized information and, with or without further psychological or chemical tests, could discuss with the patient the state of mental health as predicted by actuarial and clinical observations.

Probably most of the remedies or suggestions to be made at the time of a checkup could be actualized without further direct medical assistance. That is, the person could be involved in self-help and/or aid from family, employer, community organizations, civic groups, or nonphysician mental health workers. The array of treatment modalities, from family therapy to psychopharmacology, is increasingly impressive.

Finally, in terms of preventive service delivery, the social psychiatrist in the 1980s should attempt to contain costs by focusing on vulnerable populations. These are populations that may be more at risk for mental illness and, at the same time, require a disproportionately large amount of resources.

Therefore, as indicated in previous chapters, the social psychiatrist must give over much attention to such groups as the aged, the adults and children involved in the criminal justice system, and those who may require genetic counselling to make decisions for themselves, or for their children, both born and unborn. The latter possibility indicates how progress in the medical fields will shape the function of the psychiatrist. The state of the art now makes it reasonable to project that psychiatrists will be involved directly or indirectly in helping parents when genetic disorders (at least one of which is associated with mental retardation) are discovered and even treated in utero (Omenn, 1978).

A last issue to be discussed in delivery of service as a way of containing costs is the issue of manpower. Psychiatry, like all of medicine, will have to find ways to be less duplicative and better administered in the provision of services. At the same time there will be, perhaps, a decreasing pool of psychiatrists. Finally, by the end of the decade, a smaller pool will be available from which to select candidates for medical schools. Hence, it may be that, in this decade, manpower pinches will begin to be felt where house officers have contributed almost all the service.

In terms of demographics, the virtual certainty that 18 to 21-year-olds will decline in number during the 1980s means that there will be fewer college students. It is estimated that, compared with 1979, the numbers of 18 to 21-year-olds in 1995 will shrink by about 24% (Howe, 1979). Therefore, during the 1980s, psychiatrists will have to consider the recruitment and education of the psychiatrist and the nonpsychiatrist physician in a new manner. The development of new and effective service delivery methods will reflect much on how this recruitment and educative process evolves. Numerous factors will complicate the process, as individual and collective entitlement conflicts rage. Besides scarcity of resources and relatively decreased medical and psychiatric manpower, the 80s may bring the continued expectation that everyone is entitled to the best care available; that generally, people should work less hours and have more control over their time; and that financial rewards may not be as handsome as in previous times. All this will influence the practice of medicine. However, the very magnitude of the crisis makes it an exciting challenge. So challenging, in fact, are these sorts of issues, that as we enter the 1980s, a major societal demand is that consumers have a more active partnership and more authority with regard to how medicine meets the crisis.

THE CULTURAL CRISIS: CAN WE HELP PEOPLE TO HAVE HEALTHIER LIFE STYLES?

Culture includes the shared ideas, beliefs, and values that are conveyed from one generation to the next. The vehicle to transmit these cues in a society is communication. Among the roles of a doctor would be communication of the ideals of the society about health. As a result of consumer demands as well as professional obligation, the doctor in the 1980s will have to have more open and bilateral communication with consumers about how they can influence their own health. Presumably, each society is overcoming what it considers to be maladaptive behavior. Therefore, a society of people in the best possible health would seem to be able to develop superior communities and superior individuals. In that sense, it would be a society with less chance of producing illness.

Today there are areas of life-style that are studied enough to allow confident interpretation and communication to the general population of robust data. There are also areas that though studied, have yielded conflicting or slim data, which address areas of life-style demand important by the public. Finally, there are areas of enormous concern to the populace in terms of life-style, about which data collection or interpretation is well nigh impossible. In the midst of this entire continuum of present knowledge of life-styles is the social psychiatrist. Having roots in both biological and psychological backgrounds, the social psychiatrist has an unexcelled opportunity to help interpret and communicate about life-styles, which might ameliorate some of the misery and inequity in the society. It is a happy circumstance for social psychiatry that it has this special opportunity at a time when the public is demanding more information so that people may make informed decisions.

In this decade, more people will be persuaded to life-style changes based on their understanding of data. Substantial increases in longevity are reported for people who "exercise regularly, maintain moderate weight, eat breakfast, do not snack between meals, avoid smoking, limit liquor consumption, and sleep at least seven hours a night. A 45-year-old male who followed three or fewer of these health habits could, on the average, expect to live another 21.6 years; if he followed six or seven of them, he could expect to live another 33.1 years," (Institute of Medicine, 1978). Such data mean that informed individuals can elect to gain some control of their own longevity. The social psychiatrist wants people to elect to live longer, knowing it will mean a reduction in smoking, obesity, poor diets, drug and alcohol intake, and intemperate sedentary and sleep habits. If more people live in this manner, other crises that have been mentioned will be attenuated. For example, choosing to live in a more healthy manner should reduce the society's medical costs, and allow people to function better in artificial or natural climates.

The difficulty, of course, is that no system of education, philosophy, government, or religion has succeeded in making people follow a continent life. Recognizing the enormity of this obstacle, the social psychiatrist of the 1980s may suffer many ethical strains, as decisions must be made about the use of possible psychological manipulations or social and political actions to effect changes in behavior of adults, and mold more appropriate attitudes in children.

Actually, the interaction of doctors and consumers will force all sorts of ethical reviews. Since no data on ethics can be exhaustively conclusive, one social role of psychiatry in the 1980s may be as a broker between physicians and the public. It can be expected that, as the decade continues, there will be more formalized regulation of medical ethics.

Several states have already passed patients' rights acts. The one in Massachusetts gives patients and residents of hospitals, nursing homes, clinics, rest homes, and mental institutions the right: to receive an itemized bill; to be fully informed about risks and benefits of proposed treatment; to have privacy during treatment or care; to know when a student or trainee is involved in providing care (and to refuse to be examined, observed, or treated by students or trainees); to refuse to be a research subject or submit to examination or treatment that is for education or "informational" purposes, rather than for therapeutic reasons; to have all records and communications remain confidential; to receive prompt emergency treatment without any questions about the source of payment; to know who is responsible for their care and some pertinent facts about the attending physician, such as educational background, institutional affiliations, and financial interest in any medical facility; to obtain information about any available financial assistance and free care.

Negotiating any of these features should occasion no difficulty for any human-hearted, generous physician. However, ethical problems such as access to dialysis equipment or cadaveric parts will intensify over this decade. In the role as physicians closer to the medical model, many social psychiatrists will be called upon to take part in such deliberations. The objective data will guide such deliberations.

Therefore, the psychiatrist as counselor or consultant will sometimes be armed with data and at other times will be without it when attempting to practice the art of medicine by influencing people's life-styles. Yet at other times, the data available for participation in preventive or therapeutic efforts will be inconsistent, conflicting, and ambiguous. Thus, the physician's clinical acumen will be tested severely.

What should a social psychiatrist say about what children learn from television? Surely they learn, but the data are unclear about how, what, and why they learn (Fowles 1977). Yet should some TV content be modified or banned in the interest of public health? How should the psychiatrist relate to a pediatrician who wants to know what parents should be told about television and their children's cognitive and emotional development.

Such questions more closely resemble the traditional concern of social psychiatry during the past two decades. Much of what the social psychiatrist will do in the 1980s is an extension, of course, of these traditional concerns. The armamentarium will be stronger as new knowledge of the brain is developed (Bunney, 1979; Kolata, 1979).

Pressures of the times will place new emphasis on these traditional concerns. For instance, in the area of crime, there is a rising incidence of violent crime (murder, forcible rape, robbery, aggravated assault) by teenagers and females.

The sexual freedom achieved in the 1970s has been accompanied by an increase in teenage pregnancies, particularly in the very young adolescent. With increased female employment have come reports of increased extramarital relations of working wives. Young men come to clinics with problems related to their inability to provide sexual satisfication. The role of divorce doubled between 1963 and 1975, and the structure of the family has defied definition.

These sorts of factors present a challenge to the social psychiatrist, especially in the area of child rearing, where much preventive mental health activity is thought to take place. A society such as that of the Tarahumara Indians in Mexico is characterized by being nearly bereft of suicide, homicides, and other forms of interpersonal violence (West, 1974). Perhaps it is more than coincidence that this same society has a special tenderness, regard, and respect for children.

One last traditional concern to be mentioned is racism. This ugly reality of American life continues, as it has for hundreds of years, to inhibit the growth of democracy and freedom. As long as such injustice exists in the United States there is no way for American citizens or others to believe the rhetoric that America proclaims for itself. This is of inestimable importance since, on the one hand, it keeps Americans from feeling honest and honorable; and on the other, it retards the development of the cosmopolitan society, since the United States, a wealthy, large, and populous country, is removed from influencing others about the value of planetary citizenship. The resolution of these life-style crises will determine, to some degree, the viability of the culture, as well as the type, amount, and distribution of mental illness.

CONCLUSIONS

In looking forward to the societal, legal, and ethical issues of the 1980s, it seems that the role of social psychiatry will be to increase new types of service, to be more sensitive to consumer demands, and to work in more interdisciplinary settings.

The crises determined are ecological, sociological, and cultural. Solutions must be found to allow us to live together graciously in various artificial and cultural climates. We must contain costs, as inflation and limited resources dominate our concerns. At the same time we must attend to teaching people to choose the life-styles that will bring satisfaction and health without enraging others or causing bitterness.

Some of the considerations are not well known to social psychiatry.

Others embrace traditional concerns. No matter what is done by 1990, the crises and changes that will have been weathered will remind us of Seneca's letter about slavery (Is life-style slavery?), "Wickedness is fickle and changes frequently, not for something better but for something different."

For the social psychiatrist of the 1980s, an etymological analysis might help to define challenges and crises. Social comes from the Latin *socii*, which means allies or companions. The word psychiatry has origins in the word "suche" or soul. Thus psychiatry is the study of that without which life could not exist. Putting them together, social psychiatry is a partnership of companions or allies involved in the inquiries of those things without which life could not exist. It is a burdensome charge, but one that will make it a matchless privilege to be working in the field during these exciting and interesting times.

REFERENCES

Arthur, R.J. Success is predictable. *Mil. Med. 136:* 539-545, 1971.

Best, F. Recycling people: Work-sharing through flexible life scheduling. *The Futurist 12:* 5-17, 1978.

Bunney, W.E. Jr. (moderator). Basic and clinical studies of endorphins. *Ann. Intern. Med. 9:* 239-250, 1979.

Climate Research Board. National Academy of Sciences, *Toward a U.S. Climate Program Plan.* Washington, D.C.: 1979.

Eisenberg, L. Interfaces between medicine and psychiatry. *Comprehensive Psychiat. 20:* 1-13, 1979.

Fowles, B.R. A child and his television set. *Education and Urban Society 10:* 89-102, 1977.

Freedman, A.M.; Kaplan, H.I.; Sadock, B.J. (eds.). *Comprehensive Textbook of Psychiatry,* Second Edition Glossary, Vol. 2, Baltimore: Williams and Wilkins Co., 1975, p. 2605.

Global Atmospheric Research Program. Report of the Fourth Session of WMO Executive Committee Inter-Governmental Panel on the First GARP Experiment, Report No. 24, World Meterological Organization, International Council of Scientific Unions, Geneva, 1977, p. 63.

Howe, H. III, (Vice President for Education and Research, The Ford Foundation). *Colleges in the 1980's.* Remarks at Salem Academy and College, Winston-Salme, North Carolina, Feb. 7, 1979.

Institute of Medicine Staff Paper. *Perspectives on Health Promotion and Disease Prevention in the United States.* Washington, D.C.: National Academy of Sciences, 1979, p. vii.

Kolata, G.B. New drugs and the brain. *Science 205:* 774-776, 1979.

Omenn, G.S. Prenatal diagnosis of genetic disorders. *Science 200:* 952-958, 1978.

Pierce, C.M. Entitlement dysfunctions. *Aust. New Zealand J. Psychiat. 12:* 215-219, 1978.

Powles, J. The medicine of industrial man *Ecologist 2:* 24-36, 1972.

U.S. Committee for the Global Atmospheric Research Program. *The Global Weather Experiment - Perspectives on its Implementation and Exploitation.* Washington, D.C.: National Academy of Sciences, 1978.

West, L.J. Psychiatric problems of modern society. In *Environmental Problems in Medicine,* W.D. McKee, (ed.). Springfield: Charles C. Thomas, 1974, pp. 94-110.

ADDENDUM—CHAPTER 5

CURRENT LEGAL ISSUES AFFECTING
THE PRACTICE OF PSYCHIATRY
Jonas R. Rappeport, M.D.

The law is moving so rapidly in its attempt to clarify and resolve issues which effect our patients that what one writes today may be outdated tomorrow. Since chapter 5 was originally written, there have been several new cases relating to the Tarasoff concept and to the right to refuse treatment. There also has been legislation about confidentiality (Zurcher).

The Privacy Protection Act of 1980, passed by Congress, allowed the Department of Justice to develop guidelines for the limitations on federal law officials' use of search warrants against psychiatrists. The guidelines developed allow some protection by virtue of requiring approval of a Deputy Assistant Attorney General before such a warrant can be issued. However, there is room for abuse which would lead to an invasion of the sanctity of the consulting room (Psychiatric News, July 17, 1981, pg. 1).

The McIntosh versus Milano case was finally tried before a jury which said "...., that Dr. Michael Milano was not aware that his patient was capable of committing the 1975 murder..." (Clinical Psychiatry News, August 1981, pg. 1, 24).

In another case Lipari versus Sears, Roebuck & Co. a Federal District Court stated that there was a "Tarasoff-warning issue" to be decided by a jury after a day hospital patient, who stopped treatment one month before, murdered a total stranger and wounded several others with a shotgun his therapist knew he owned. [(This case has subsequently been settled) (Lipari vs Sears, Roebuck & Co. -497 F. Suppl 185, 1980).] However, in a Maryland case, the Appeals Court said there was no basis for requiring a warning by the psychiatrist due to the state's statutory psychiatrist-patient privilege (Shaw versus Glickman 415 A 2d. 625, 1980). Courts have varied in their opinions so a majority position is not yet clear.

The issue of the right to refuse treatment has been quite active. There have been several hearings on the Rennie case. The latest

143

Rennie decision by the Federal District Court has essentially placed the responsibility for review of the patient's refusal back into the hands of the hospital superintendent without all of the procedures required by the lower court judge (79-2576-2577 U.S.D.C. 3rd Cir., July 9, 1981). A new case, Rogers versus Okin, in Massachusetts has been heard at several levels and is currently scheduled to be heard before the U.S. Supreme Court in December 1981. In essence, in this case, the Circuit Court of Appeals agreed that patients had a right to refuse treatment if competent and not dangerous to staff or other patients, but they might have to then be discharged, etc. That court recognized that the patient's health could be harmed by allowing him to refuse treatment. However, they continued to see antipsychotic medication as "mind-altering" as had the lower court (Rogers vs Okin, 79-1648 & 79-1649 1st. Cir., Nov. 25, 1980).

Some cases have involved money awards against the treating and supervising physicians and spoken of the least restrictive form of treatment possible being utilized for objecting patients. These cases, Scott versus Plank (N.J.) and Romeo versus Youngbreg (Pa.), have been heard by District Courts of Appeals, 80-1314, 1315, 1596 (Feb. 5, 1981) and 80-1429. The courts eventually seem reluctant to place monetary demands on physicians who were not responsible for understaffing, etc.; however, such "excuses" are wearing thin.

There have been several other cases on both the Right to Treatment and the Right to Refuse Treatment. Since the Supreme Court will render an opinion within the next year, it seems useless to mention every case. Hopefully the court will render a broad-based opinion, which will then give us the guidance we need.

INDEX